BASALT REGIONAL LIBRARY DISTRICT

99 MIDLAND AVENUE
BASALT CO 81621
927-4311

BASALT REGIONAL LIBRARY DISTRICT

1 44 0000242

D0578297

613.2 DIE
American Academy of
  Pediatrics guide to your
  child's nutrition   23 85

JY -7 '99	DATE DUE	
NOV 1 8 '99		
MAR 3 1 '00		
JE -8 02		
NO -6 02		
NO 29 '02		
AUG 1 3 2003		
SE 1 8 '03		
NO 6 03		
JAN 2 6 2004		
MAR 3 2004		

**CHILDCARE BOOKS FROM THE
AMERICAN ACADEMY OF PEDIATRICS**

**The American Academy of Pediatrics
Guide to Your Child's Symptoms**

Your Baby's First Year

**Caring for Your Baby and Young Child
Birth to Age 5**

**Caring for Your School-Age Child
Ages 5 to 12**

**Caring for Your Adolescent
Ages 12 to 21**

AMERICAN ACADEMY OF PEDIATRICS

GUIDE TO YOUR CHILD'S NUTRITION

AMERICAN ACADEMY OF PEDIATRICS

GUIDE TO YOUR CHILD'S NUTRITION

Making Peace at the Table
and Building Healthy
Eating Habits for Life

EDITORS

William H. Dietz, M.D., Ph.D., F.A.A.P.
Director, Division of Nutrition and Physical Activity
National Center for Chronic Disease Prevention and
Health Promotion
Centers for Disease Control and Prevention
Atlanta, Georgia

Loraine Stern, M.D., F.A.A.P.
Associate Clinical Professor
Department of Pediatrics
University of California at Los Angeles
and in private practice, general pediatrics
Los Angeles, California

Villard
New York

Basalt Regional Library
99 Midland Avenue
Basalt CO 81621

Copyright © 1999 by American Academy of Pediatrics

All rights reserved under International and Pan-American Copyright Conventions. Published in the United States by Villard Books, a division of Random House, Inc., New York, and simultaneously in Canada by Random House of Canada Limited, Toronto.

VILLARD BOOKS is a registered trademark of Random House, Inc.

ISBN: 0-375-50187-8

Random House website address: www.atrandom.com

Printed in the United States of America on acid-free paper

98765432

First Edition

This book is dedicated to all the people who recognize that children are our greatest inspiration in the present and our greatest hope for the future.

From the Editors
We dedicate this book to the children who have taught us what we really know and the parents who have helped them teach us.

Dr. Dietz thanks his wife, Nan Dietz, for her support.

Dr. Stern thanks her husband, Jack Nides, for his support and her stepdaughter, Tina Nides, the mother of her writing career.

Co-Editors
William H. Dietz, M.D., Ph.D.
Loraine Stern, M.D.

AAP Board of Directors Reviewer
Donald Cook, M.D.

American Academy of Pediatrics
Executive Director
Joe M. Sanders, Jr., M.D.

Associate Executive Director
Roger F. Suchyta, M.D.

Director, Department of Communications
Linda L. Martin

Director, Division of Public Education
Lisa R. Reisberg

Project Manager, Division of Public Education
Mark T. Grimes

Project Coordinator, Division of Public Education
Kate Larson

Reviewers and Contributors
Susan Baker, M.D.
Miriam Bar-on, M.D.
William Cochran, M.D.
Betty Crase, I.B.C.L.C.
Evelyn Eisenstein, M.D.
Marianne Felice, M.D.
Carlos Flores, M.D.
Lawrence Gartner, M.D.
Michael Georgieff, M.D.
Elizabeth Gleghorn, M.D.
Peter Gorski, M.D.
Marc Jacobson, M.D.
Tom Jaksic, M.D.
Desmond Kelly, M.D.

Nancy Krebs, M.D.
Annette Lansford, M.D.
Greg Prazar, M.D.
Peter Rappo, M.D.
Carol Redell, M.D.
Barbara Reid, M.D.
Robert Rothbaum, M.D.
Robert Squires, M.D.
Susan Tully, M.D.
John Udall, M.D.
Robert Wood, M.D.

Acknowledgments
Editorial production by DSH Editorial, Inc.,
a division of G.S. Sharpe Communications, Inc.

Editorial Director
Genell J. Subak-Sharpe, M.S.

Managing Editor
Rosemary Perkins

Writers
Densie P. Webb, R.D., Ph.D.
Rosemary Perkins

Copy Editor
Mary P. Willard

Designers
Tanya Krawciw
Peter Lukic
Danusia Wasylkiwskij

Illustrators
Wendy Wray
Briar Lee Mitchell

Secretarial Support
Debbie Carney

Technical Assistance
Mary Claire Walsh

Guide to Your Child's Nutrition

PLEASE NOTE

The information contained in this book is intended to complement, not substitute for, the advice of your child's pediatrician. Before starting any treatment or program affecting your child's health and nutrition, you should consult your own pediatrician, who can discuss your child's individual needs with you and counsel you about symptoms and treatment.

The information and advice in this book apply equally to children of both sexes. We have elected to alternate the use of he and she instead of using a single gender pronoun or the awkward he/she construction. When a problem is more common in one sex than the other, it is so indicated. Otherwise, you should assume that either gender can be equally affected, even though only one is referred to in the text.

FOREWORD

The American Academy of Pediatrics *Guide to Your Child's Nutrition* is the latest in a series of books for parents developed by the American Academy of Pediatrics.

The American Academy of Pediatrics is an organization of 53,000 primary care pediatricians, pediatric medical subspecialists, and pediatric surgical specialists dedicated to the health, safety, and well-being of infants, children, adolescents, and young adults. This book is part of the Academy's ongoing education efforts to provide parents and caregivers with high-quality information on a broad spectrum of children's health issues.

What distinguishes this book from many other reference books in bookstores and on library shelves is that it has been written and extensively reviewed by members of the American Academy of Pediatrics. Under the direction of our two co-editors, the initial material was developed with the assistance of more than 20 reviewers and contributors. Because medical information about children's health is constantly changing, every effort has been made to ensure that this book contains the most up-to-date information available.

It is the Academy's hope that this book will become an invaluable resource and reference guide for parents. We believe it is the best source of information on matters of children's health and well-being. We are confident readers will find the book extremely valuable, and we encourage readers to use it in concert with the advice and counsel of their own pediatricians, who will provide individual guidance and assistance on issues related to the health of their children.

Joe M. Sanders, Jr., M.D.
Executive Director

AMERICAN ACADEMY OF PEDIATRICS

GUIDE TO YOUR CHILD'S NUTRITION

Peace at the Table:
The Whys and Hows of Nurturance

One of our favorite cartoons is "Baby Blues," by Rick Kirkman and Jerry Scott. A young couple have two children, a preschooler and an infant. In one strip, the preschooler climbs up on a stool next to her mother and asks, "What are you cooking?"

"Chicken and rice," her mother answers.

The child screws up her face, throws herself on the floor, and writhes, yelling, "Bleah! Yuk! Gaak!"

In the last box, she lies quietly on the floor and asks, "What's that taste like?"

What we hope this book will do, among other things, is help you to be calm and effectual when faced with situations such as this.

> *Feeding children should be a shared responsibility: "The parent is responsible for WHAT; the child is responsible for HOW MUCH and even WHETHER."*
>
> —Ellyn Satter, author of *How to Get Your Kid to Eat—But Not Too Much*

Meals: Time to Relax and Enjoy

"Nurture" means "to care for" and "to feed." As we nurture our children, we often allow food to become an indicator of how well we are doing our job. As a result, food turns into a measure of how much our children love us and obey us, rather than a source of energy and nutrients. Food becomes emotionally charged, and mealtimes are a source of anxiety and tension rather than opportunities to relax, interact, and enjoy one another.

What we offer children and what they eat have a great deal to do with their health and growth. But whether they actually eat what we serve depends on more than what we choose to lay before them. Their own tastes and preferences, their moods, and—most important—what they learn from people around them in subtle and not-so-subtle ways determine what and how much they eat.

The title of this book includes "peace at the table." Peace is best maintained by wise administrators who know when to intervene and when to hold back, not by a police state. If you turn into "food police," our experience is that you may provoke conflict and make the situation worse. Remember your respective roles: As parents, you are responsible for offering a healthful variety of foods. Your children are responsible for deciding what and how much they want to eat from what they are offered.

Offer Wholesome Choices, Then Stand Aside

Children will not become ill or suffer permanently if they refuse a meal or two, but parents sometimes act as though youngsters might shrivel up and die. Parents' fears and concessions have produced toddlers who will eat only white foods such as milk, macaroni, white bread, and potatoes, or children who take no food other than milk, or parents who collapse in tears at every mealtime while their toddler rules the family from her booster seat. All of these situations eventually resolve; all of them can be prevented. With infants and young children, your job is to offer wholesome food choices and then step back.

Lois, the mother of a patient, told Dr. Loraine Stern the following story: Lois's sister and brother-in-law took off for a long weekend, leaving Kristin, their 8-year-old daughter, with Lois. When they dropped Kristin off, they also left a long list of what she would and wouldn't eat. Lois accepted the list and wished her sister and brother-in-law a good time.

That evening at dinnertime, Kristin asked, "What are we having?"

When Lois told her, she screwed up her face and said, "I don't like that."

"Gee, I'm sorry," Lois said. "You don't have to eat it if you don't want to."

Kristin left the main course on her plate, although she picked a little at the side dishes while she pouted. Lois paid no attention and took Kristin's plate away when everyone was through. Kristin probably went to bed a little hungry. However, the next morning, because she was hungry, she relished what was served for breakfast. She made no more complaints and ate well the entire weekend. Of course, we're sure she went back to her pickiness with her parents when they returned.

After Kelly, a colleague of Dr. William Dietz, found herself making a separate main course for her 4-year-old every time she cooked something he didn't like, she promised herself this would not happen with her next child. So when 3-year-old Colleen turned up her nose at the fish the rest of the family was eating, Kelly said, "You don't have to eat it. I'll just put it in the refrigerator and you can have it later if you want."

When bedtime arrived, Colleen said, "I think I'd better eat that fish or I'll get hungry."

This tactic really works.

Emotions Complicate Nutrition

Parents of young children worry mostly about whether their children are eating enough of the right foods. Among older children and adolescents, however, the most important issues are usually obesity and eating disorders, such as anorexia and bulimia. Early experiences, interactions within the family around foods, the influence of peers, the media, and lifestyles that reduce the time children spend eating with the family all probably contribute to these diseases. In addition, a teenager who is preoccupied with weight and body image may both literally and symbolically slam the door when worried parents try to discuss issues of food and weight. Every pediatrician has the experience of seeing unexpected tears on a teenager's cheeks when the subject of weight arises during a checkup. In these families, everyone is upset: parents, because everything they do seems to make matters worse; adolescents, because they want their parents' help, but only on their own terms.

This situation is not very different from food issues with younger children. The nutrients in food are only part of the problem. Emotional, behavioral, and psychological issues are equally important.

Nutrition: A Long-Range Issue

In this book, we emphasize healthful food choices and the Food Guide Pyramid, but we do not emphasize rigid fat- and calorie-counting. Nutrition is a long-range issue, and one day or one week does not make or break good health. Rather, we want you to develop a perspective on how to feed your children a wholesome diet and maintain a healthful lifestyle, how to allow for individual styles and preferences, and how to make shared mealtimes enjoyable as well as stress- and guilt-free.

This book reflects not only the writers' and editors' experience and opinion, but also information reviewed by many experts. Although we have included personal anecdotes from our practices, this book represents the consensus of the 53,000 pediatricians of North and South America who are members of the American Academy of Pediatrics. Members include pediatricians, pediatric medical subspecialists, and pediatric surgical specialists.

The *Guide to Your Child's Nutrition* is designed to be useful at various points in your children's lives and to help solve particular problems that may arise. Because we know it may not be read straight through, some sections may be repetitious. This is deliberate. We want to make sure that a parent consulting us from time to time will not miss important points that are covered in other parts of the book.

Peace, and *bon appétit!*

William H. Dietz, M.D., Ph.D., F.A.A.P.
Loraine Stern, M.D., F.A.A.P.
Editors

CHAPTER 1

What's Best for My Newborn?

When Laura and Jim Hawkins brought baby Emily home from the hospital, they were both overjoyed and overwhelmed. "We were absolutely delighted to finally have a baby," Laura recalls, "but neither of us knew anything about infant care. Since I planned to breastfeed, I figured I'd instinctively know what to do. It didn't take long for reality to set in!" Nurses at the hospital helped Laura start breastfeeding, and showed her such babycare basics as diapering and bathing. But in just two days, the Hawkinses were on their own at home. "For weeks we called our pediatrician almost daily with questions," Laura recounts.

Like many new parents, you're probably eager to do what's "right." We want to stress at the outset that you're embarking on one of life's greatest and most rewarding adventures—namely, parenthood. Usually, there is no right or wrong way; instead, it's a matter of deciding what works best for you and your baby. So relax. Enjoy getting to know your new baby and trust your own sense of what's right for you.

Not surprisingly, many of these questions dealt with Emily's diet. "How often should I feed her?" "How can I tell whether she's getting enough milk?" "Should I give her supplemental formula 'just in case'?" "Does she need extra iron and vitamins?" "What about water?" "Her stools are runny and yellowish. Does she have diarrhea?" "I have a bad cold. Is it safe for me to breastfeed?" "What should I do if I'm unable to nurse for a few days?"

Common Concerns

Many if not most new parents have similar concerns. In fact, parents ask pediatricians more questions about how and what to feed their babies than about any other aspect of early childcare.

Although this book is intended to answer the most frequently asked of these questions, it's important to remember that no two babies are exactly alike: What's good for your baby isn't necessarily good for your sister's or your neighbor's. Your pediatrician is your best source of advice about what's best for your baby, and you should not hesitate to discuss any concerns with him or her.

Decisions, Decisions

Even before your baby's birth, you need to decide how you want to feed her: Will you feed your baby breastmilk or formula? The American Academy of Pediatrics, the American Dietetic Association, and other organizations concerned with health and nutrition advocate breastfeeding for most women, and a growing number of American women plan to nurse.

The American Academy of Pediatrics has always advocated breastfeeding as the best way to nourish babies. Breastfeeding is best for the health of babies and mothers alike. It is economical and convenient.

In new and even stronger guidelines, the Academy encourages mothers to breastfeed exclusively for the first 6 months (about the time your baby's diet begins to include solid foods), and to continue breastfeeding for at least 12 months or as long as baby and mother want to continue.

A survey found that 80 to 90 percent of pregnant women wanted to breastfeed, but in actual practice, only about 60 percent of American mothers start nursing. Although this figure is lower than we'd like it to be, it's a marked improvement over the all-time low of 26.5 percent in 1970.

The guidelines recommend that health insurers cover necessary services and supplies. They emphasize the importance of providing workplace facilities where working mothers can pump milk to save for their babies.

Breastfeeding has many advantages (see The Special Health Benefits of Breastfeeding, p. 9), but there are instances in which it is not possible: for example, when a baby has a condition such as classic galactosemia, also known as GALT deficiency, which is a rare, inborn inability to digest the sugar in milk. A mother may also be advised not to breastfeed when she is HIV-positive or has a serious disorder, such as hepatitis B, that could be passed in the breastmilk, or takes medication that might harm her baby (see Why Some Women Should Not Breastfeed, p. 14). Personal factors may make nursing impossible, and some women and/or their partners simply are not comfortable with the idea or they harbor mistaken notions about what it entails (see Common Myths About Breastfeeding, p. 19). At any rate, you should talk over the pros and cons of breastfeeding with your obstetrician and pediatrician well before your due date. Learn as much as possible about breastfeeding, and make the best decision for your baby and yourself.

Even though breastfeeding is a natural function, most women need help in getting started. Prenatal classes often include breastfeeding instructions. Some doctors and maternity centers have lactation consultants—specially trained nurses or other health professionals—who teach the basics of breastfeeding. Maternity nurses also help teach new mothers. Unfortunately, the trend toward 24- to 48-hour hospital stays following delivery often doesn't allow enough time to ensure that all is going smoothly before going home. If problems do arise after you leave the hospital, your pediatrician can help you or may recommend a lactation consultant. Many lactation consultants make home visits. There are also support groups for nursing mothers (see Health and Nutrition Resources, Appendix VI).

Getting Started

The offspring of any mammal instinctively seeks out a nipple and begins suckling within minutes of being born. Similarly, most human babies are alert and eager to suckle shortly after birth, provided there are no problems. Mothers who nurse while still in the delivery room typically describe a deep sense of pleasure and satisfaction. The earlier breastfeeding starts, the easier it is for mother and baby. However, if the first attempt is delayed, breastfeeding can still be initiated successfully later. Olfactory bonding—through which a baby learns to recognize his own mother's scent—develops while the mother holds her baby, even if he is not suckling.

Regardless of when the first feeding takes place, you may need help positioning your baby comfortably and getting him to "latch on" properly. To do this, with your baby lying on his side, bring

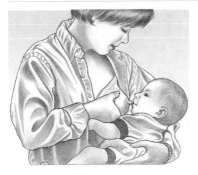

Figure 1

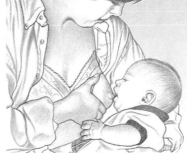

Figure 2

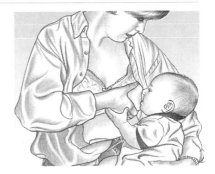

Figure 3

his head up to your breast until his nose is level with your nipple (Figure 1). Hold your baby with one arm and use the other hand to support the breast. Gently stroke his lips with your nipple or finger to stimulate his rooting reflex and interest in nursing (Figure 2). You also may try squeezing out a few drops of milk, then lightly brushing the nipple against your baby's lower lip; this will further stimulate his desire to nurse and prompt him to open his mouth wide. When his mouth is fully open, quickly bring your baby to the breast with his lips around the areola

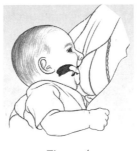

Figure 4

and the nipple deep in his mouth (Figure 3). This allows your baby to latch on and begin suckling. Make sure your baby's face is not at an angle to your nipple, but facing straight on to your breast. Your baby's chest and abdomen also should be facing directly toward your chest and abdomen. His neck should be straight and not turned.

It's important to position the nipple far back in your baby's mouth so that it touches the roof of her mouth and she is able to compress the areola, which contains the milk sinuses, as she suckles (Figure 4). If she latches on to only the nipple, milk can dribble out the side of her mouth. In addition, sucking on the nipple alone can make it sore and cracked. You'll soon be able to feel whether your baby is suckling properly; in the beginning, check that the nipple and most of the areola are inside your baby's mouth, with her nose and chin just touching the breast and the lips relaxed. Her jaws should move up and down, her ears should wiggle as she suckles, and she should swallow after every few sucks. If you have continuing pain, take your baby off the breast

▶ **NURSING CRAMPS**

For days or weeks after delivery, many women have cramping pain in the abdomen at the start of each feeding. This is because nursing stimulates the release of hormones that help shrink the uterus back to its normal size.

Almost all nursing mothers describe breastfeeding as a highly pleasurable experience, but to make it so, you need to find a position that is comfortable for both you and your baby. Experiment with the following positions until you find what works best for you at various times.

Lying down. Both you and your baby lie on your sides facing each other. Rest your baby's head in the crook of your arm with a pillow at his back for support. Place a pillow under your head and another behind your back so you can be at the correct angle for your baby to latch on. A pillow between your knees is also comfortable. Women recovering from a cesarean delivery often find this the most comfortable position; it's also good for night feedings. After the feedings, put your baby back in his crib. It's the safest place for him to sleep.

Cradle hold. Sit in a comfortable chair or in bed with pillows tucked behind your back, under your arm on the nursing side, and on your lap to support your baby. Position your baby on his side with his tummy close to yours, his head cradled in the crook of your arm with his face next to your breast, his back resting along your forearm, and his bottom supported by your hand. In this and other positions, he should be able to latch on without turning his head. If your baby is very small or has a weak sucking reflex, try supporting the back of his head with your other hand rather than placing it in the crook of your elbow. (This is sometimes called the modified cradle or transitional hold.)

Clutch, side, or football hold. Sit in a comfortable chair (a roomy rocker is ideal) with a pillow on your lap to bring your baby up level with your breast. Position him with his legs under your arm and his head resting on your hand. If your arm gets tired, support it on a pillow or your thigh (bend your knee and place your foot on a stool or low table). The side position works especially well if you have large breasts or flat nipples, or after a cesarean section.

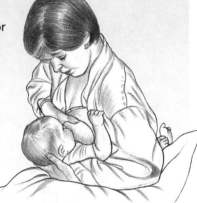

and reposition her. If your breasts are large and your baby's nose is buried, draw her bottom and legs closer to your midsection and lift your breast up a bit from underneath to let your baby breathe from the sides of her nose as she nurses.

When your baby stops nursing, gently break the suction by inserting a finger in the corner of her mouth, letting in some air and encouraging your baby to let go. To prevent injury to the nipple, do not pull your baby off the breast while she is still suckling and tightly attached.

Breastfeeding and Intelligence
Several studies of children's development reveal some intriguing findings about the relationship between breastfeeding and intelligence. Children

 THE SPECIAL HEALTH BENEFITS OF BREASTFEEDING

Pediatricians and nutrition experts agree that breastmilk is the ideal food for newborns and young babies. It's also inexpensive, and breastfeeding has emotional and physical benefits for the mother. Here are some of the reasons:

- Breastmilk is uniquely tailored to meet all your baby's nutritional needs for about the first 6 months of life. Its composition changes as your baby's needs change. For example, during the first few days the breasts secrete colostrum, which is especially rich in antibodies to protect against infections. It also contains substances that get your baby's digestive system working.

- Babies can digest breastmilk more easily than formula.

- According to several researchers, breastfed babies have fewer allergies, intestinal upsets, ear infections, and other common childhood problems than their formula-fed counterparts. If there is a family history of asthma, eczema, hayfever, or other allergies, breastfeeding is especially important in reducing allergy symptoms. The longer you nurse, the better.

- The benefits of breastfeeding appear to extend beyond infancy. Studies show that children who were breastfed have lower rates of diabetes, asthma, and certain other chronic illnesses—benefits that tend to persist into adulthood.

- Breastfeeding is cheaper and more convenient than formula.

- Breastfed babies adapt more readily to new foods when solids are introduced.

- A baby's suckling prompts the release of oxytocin, a pituitary hormone that, in addition to triggering the flow of breastmilk, causes the uterus to contract and regain its pre-pregnancy size more quickly.

- Women who breastfeed have lower rates of certain types of breast and ovarian cancers and fewer hip fractures later in life.

who had been nourished on breastmilk did slightly but consistently better on standard tests in school than those who were fed formula. The longer they were breastfed, the better they did. What's more, the advantages persisted well beyond early childhood. The breastfed children were more likely to complete high school, irrespective of their family income, education, and standard of living, among other factors. Thus, breastfed babies appear not only to be healthier but also to do better in school.

Nutritional factors in breastmilk, a lower rate of illnesses, and psychological effects may also help explain the better performance seen in breastfed children.

Vitamins for Breastfed Babies

Breastmilk provides sufficient amounts of vitamins except, possibly, for vitamin D in some specific cases. Vitamin D promotes the absorption of calcium and is needed to build healthy bones and teeth. Babies who are not regularly exposed to sunlight, who have dark skin, and who are dressed heavily when outside may not get enough of this vitamin. Your pediatrician may prescribe a vitamin D supplement for your breastfed infant. Commercial formulas are usually fortified with vitamin D and other vitamins to ensure that babies get enough of these essential nutrients.

A mother who follows a vegan diet, which excludes all foods of animal origin, should talk to her pediatrician about her baby's vitamin needs. A vegan diet lacks both vitamin D and vitamin B_{12}. A deficiency of vitamin B_{12} in an infant's diet can lead to anemia and abnormalities of the nervous system.

Bottle Feeding

Although no infant formula exactly duplicates breastmilk—and experts agree that mother's milk is best—the reality is that 85 percent of babies in the United States, including many who are breastfed, are given formula for at least some feedings. In some instances, mothers use formula because they choose not to or cannot breastfeed. Formula is also used to give Mom an occasional break or, less commonly, to supplement inadequate production of breastmilk. There are also medical conditions that prevent breastfeeding (see Why Some Women Should Not Breastfeed, p. 14).

A baby may have a problem that requires a special formula, either as the primary food or as a supplement to breastmilk. For example, premature or low-birth-weight babies may need special formulas to supply the extra energy and nutrients they need for growth. In these small babies, too, the sucking reflex may not be fully developed, in which case they will be fed with a special tube or by bottle. Still, a premature infant can benefit from the anti-

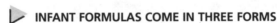

INFANT FORMULAS COME IN THREE FORMS

■ The ready-to-use types are the most convenient—all you need to do is pour them into a clean bottle—but they are also the most expensive.

■ Concentrated liquid formulas are mixed with an equal amount of water; these are not as costly as the ready-to-use type, but you must make sure that the water is clean.

■ Powdered formulas are the least expensive; they also require the most preparation.

bodies and other unique components of breast-milk. Mothers of premature and other high-risk infants are usually encouraged to express their breastmilk, which may be fortified with the additional nutrients needed and fed to her baby. Then when the baby is ready to breastfeed directly from mother, the switch can be made.

Infants from highly allergic families may react to certain foods the mother eats that then pass into the breastmilk, such as the protein from cow's milk

▶ PRACTICAL BOTTLE-FEEDING TIPS

- Bottle feeding can be a warm, loving experience: Cuddle your baby closely, gaze into her eyes, and coo and talk to her. Never prop the bottle and let your baby feed alone; not only will you miss the opportunity to bond with her while she feeds, but there's also a danger she'll choke or the bottle will slip out of position. This practice also increases the risk of ear infections. We do not recommend devices to hold a bottle in a baby's mouth—they could be dangerous.

- Although some babies will drink a bottle straight from the refrigerator, most prefer milk warmed to room temperature. You can warm a bottle by holding it under a running hot-water faucet or placing it in a bowl of hot water for a few minutes. Sprinkle a few drops on your wrist; it should feel lukewarm. If it's too warm, wait for it to cool a bit and test again.

Note: NEVER warm a bottle of formula or breastmilk in the microwave. The bottle itself may feel cool, while the liquid inside can be too hot. Microwaving also heats unevenly. Even though a few drops sprinkled on your wrist may feel okay, some of the formula or breastmilk may be scalding. Also, the composition of breastmilk may change.

- Make sure the nipple hole is the right size. If your baby seems to be gagging or gulping too fast, the nipple hole may be too large. Similarly, if your baby is sucking hard and seems frustrated, the hole may be too small.

- Try different nipple shapes to see which your baby prefers. There is no "correct" shape.

- Angle the bottle so your baby isn't sucking in air. Burp your baby a couple of times during the course of a feeding.

- Encourage your partner to give your baby a bottle now and then, perhaps one of the late-night feedings. This not only allows you some extra rest, but it also fosters father-infant bonding.

- Don't let your baby fall asleep sucking on a bottle of milk, especially if she is beginning to cut teeth. Milk pooled in your baby's mouth can cause serious tooth decay, known as nursing-bottle caries. After feeding and before putting your baby to sleep, gently wipe any milk residues from her gums. If she needs to suck herself to sleep, give her a pacifier instead of a bottle.

- Repeated sterilization may distort nipple openings. Test to make sure milk flow through the nipple is adequate.

or cheese, or from eggs, seafood, and nuts. Breastfeeding mothers can help prevent allergies in their infants by avoiding such foods while nursing. In rare cases, such as certain metabolic diseases, a baby may not be able to tolerate breastmilk, in which case a special formula will be needed. A physical abnormality that makes it difficult for a baby to suckle normally, such as a cleft palate, may make breastfeeding impossible (see p. 18).

There are many kinds of infant formulas; most are based on cow's milk, but there are also several formulas available for babies who cannot tolerate cow's milk. Regular cow's and goat's milk, as well as canned condensed or evaporated milk, should not be given during the first year of life. Young babies cannot digest the protein in cow's milk. Regular cow's milk also doesn't have enough iron and other vitamins or the right amounts of the minerals that are essential for proper growth and development. A child may also lose blood through the stools, because cow's milk can damage the intestine.

What's in It for My Baby?

Although no formulas on the market even come close to matching the hundreds of known ingredients in breastmilk, most provide a comparable balance of fat, protein, and sugar. Formulas are also supplemented with various vitamins and minerals, especially calcium, iron, and vitamins C, D, and K. Should you choose not to breastfeed, your pediatrician can advise which formula is most suitable for your baby. Sometimes you may need to switch formulas if your baby is ill.

Regardless of which formula you use, it's critical that you prepare it according to instructions. It is especially important not to add more or less water than recommended. Families who are short of money may be tempted to add extra water to make

the formula go farther. Formulas are designed to provide the energy (about 20 calories per ounce) and nutrients that a baby needs for proper growth. If the formula is too weak, your baby will be underfed and may have stunted growth and nutritional deficiencies. Formula that's too strong can also be dangerous. Not adding enough water can result in dehydration, kidney problems, and other potentially serious disorders.

Sterilizing and Warming Bottles

Parents and pediatricians today are not as concerned with sterilizing bottles and water as they were a generation ago. But many are having second thoughts in light of recent reports of contaminated city water supplies and increased concern over food safety. For starters, always wash your hands before handling baby bottles or feeding your baby. If you use disposable plastic bottle liners and ready-to-use formula, you still need to make sure the nipples are clean. Scrub them in hot, soapy water, then rinse to get rid of all traces of soap; some experts recommend boiling them for 5 to 10 minutes. Always wash and thoroughly rinse and dry the top of the formula can before you open it; also make sure the can opener, mixing cups, jars, spoons, and other equipment are clean.

If you use regular glass bottles and concentrated or powdered formula, you must make sure that the bottles and water added to the formula are germ-free. If you don't want to boil the bottles, you can put them, along with mixing cups and other equipment used to prepare the formula, in a dishwasher that uses heated water and has a hot drying cycle. Or you can wash the bottles in hot, soapy water and rinse thoroughly. This alone should kill most germs; any that do survive the washing can be killed by putting the empty bottles in an oven set at 250°F for 20 minutes or in a microwave oven set on medium for 4 minutes.

In general, tap water that comes from a municipal system is safe for older babies and children. But for the first month or two, it's a good idea to boil water for at least 5 minutes. Or you can use sterile bottled water. There is no need to sterilize bottles after your baby is about 3 months old.

If you elect to boil your bottles and don't want to invest in a sterilizer, use a large covered pot. There are two general methods:

- Place the empty bottles, along with the measuring cup and other equipment used to make the formula, in a large pot, fill with water to completely cover all items, and boil for 20 minutes. When the bottles are cool enough, either cover them and put them away, or fill with breastmilk or formula, refrigerate, and use within 48 hours. (Breastmilk in bottles can be refrigerated for at least 12 hours.)
- Fill the bottles with breastmilk or formula, loosely screw on the caps, and place the bottles in a pot large enough so that they can stand upright. Add a few inches of water, cover the pot, and boil for 25 minutes. Tighten caps, refrigerate, and use within 48 hours.

Supplemental Bottles

Many breastfeeding mothers use an occasional bottle of expressed, frozen breastmilk or formula because they need to be away from the baby. In unusual cases, a pediatrician may recommend a combination of breastfeeding and formula if the mother is returning to work, or if she is ill or exhausted. It is commonly—though often wrongly—thought that supplemental bottles are given because the mother does not have enough milk. As stressed earlier, the vast majority of mothers produce more than enough milk to meet their babies' needs, even for twins. When there appears to be a problem of supply-and-demand, your pediatrician may encourage you to see a lactation consultant.

> ▷ **DISCARD ANY LEFTOVERS**
>
> A note of caution: If your baby does not drink the entire bottle, discard what's left over. Germs and enzymes from your baby's mouth can enter the bottle and spoil the milk.

If supplemental bottles are given for the sake of convenience, experts advise waiting until your baby is 3 or 4 weeks old. This allows time for your milk supply to become well established, and for you and your baby to get used to breastfeeding. Don't be surprised if your baby doesn't immediately take to a bottle. To obtain the benefits of human milk, it is best if you express your breastmilk and store it for bottle feeding as needed. Expressing breastmilk also helps maintain your milk supply. Formula can also be fed while you continue breastfeeding as often as possible. Use the formula your pediatrician recommends.

Breastfeeding Problem Solving

Many women breastfeed with nary a problem, but others may encounter difficulties. Fortunately, most problems are easily solved. If the measures outlined below don't work, talk to your doctor or a lactation consultant.

INVERTED OR FLAT NIPPLES. Inverted or flat nipples do not preclude nursing and, in many cases, can be corrected. Your obstetrician may recommend breast shells worn during the last trimester, with the time gradually increasing to 4 to 6 hours a day. After your baby is born, the nipples will respond to suckling. Other devices are sometimes recommended, but they often don't work and can make the breasts sore and promote infection. Nipple shields are not recommended.

ENGORGEMENT (OVERFILLED BREASTS). This usually occurs in the first few days of breastfeeding or when you cut back on nursing, resulting in over-filled breasts. Engorgement usually can be prevented by frequent nursing and draining the breasts. Make sure your baby is suckling properly. If your breasts are producing more milk than your baby can consume, you may need to express the excess before he latches on. If pain is hindering your milk flow (letdown), taking a warm shower or applying a warm compress before nursing may help. Some women find cold compresses or ice packs provide more relief. Occasional use of a breastpump may also help. Experiment to find what works best for you, but above all, don't cut back on your breastfeeding; this will worsen the problem. Regular, frequent breastfeeding is the best way to prevent and relieve engorgement.

CRACKED OR SORE NIPPLES. First, try to find out the cause. Most often, it turns out that the nipple is incorrectly placed in the baby's mouth. If the soreness develops in the first few weeks of breastfeeding, check to make sure your baby is latching on properly, with most of the areola in his mouth. He may possibly be chewing or gumming on the nipple, or perhaps his lower lip is turned inward, which can lead to soreness and even cracking.

To heal the nipples, try expressing a few drops of colostrum or mature milk and rubbing it gen-

▷ **WHY SOME WOMEN SHOULD NOT BREASTFEED**

Doctors advise women not to breastfeed under the following conditions:

■ If they have certain infectious diseases, a positive HIV test or AIDS, human T-cell leukemia virus (HTLV) infection, or untreated tuberculosis, that could be passed on to their babies.

■ If they must take medications—such as cyclosporine, antithyroid medications, or drugs that suppress the immune system—that pass into the breastmilk and are harmful to babies. Most medicines prescribed by your physician are likely to be safe for breastfed babies, but it's best to ask him or her to check them. If you're breastfeeding, always check with your pediatrician before taking any nonprescription, herbal, or folk or natural remedies.

■ If they use marijuana, cocaine, heroin, amphetamines, or other illicit/recreational drugs.

■ If their breasts lack enough glandular tissue to make milk. This is very rare, and is unrelated to breast size—women with small breasts can produce as much milk as large-breasted women.

■ Women who have chronic or debilitating medical conditions may be advised not to breastfeed. Some doctors think that women with silicone breast implants should not breastfeed, but there is no evidence that children are harmed by implants.

tly into the sore area. Allow the milk to dry on the nipples. Wash them with plain water and avoid using soap, which promotes cracking by removing protective skin oils. Don't use ointments or creams unless specifically recommended by your doctor. Ultrapurified anhydrous lanolin may promote healing and does not need to be removed from the nipples before nursing.

POOR MILK LETDOWN. Letdown is the automatic release of milk stored in breast tissue into the milk ducts, allowing it to flow more easily into your baby's mouth. Suckling stimulates the letdown reflex; infrequent nursing or a poor latch-on to the breast can hinder it. Stress, pain, fatigue, anxiety, nicotine, alcohol, and certain medications are among the many factors that can inhibit letdown. In most instances, you can solve letdown problems with frequent nursing and proper positioning of your baby on the breast. You should also try to reduce stress and avoid alcohol and caffeine. Before breastfeeding, try massaging your breasts, gently rubbing your nipples, applying warm compresses, or taking a warm shower. When using a breastpump, mental images can also trigger release of the hormone (oxytocin) that prompts letdown; picture your baby nursing. In some women, just hearing a baby cry triggers letdown. If none of these tactics works, ask your doctor or consultant for advice.

LEAKY BREASTS. Leaking is most common in the early weeks of breastfeeding, but it's not unusual for it to continue for weeks or even months. Sometimes leaking occurs when you're not breastfeeding. Also, some women leak without a letdown, just from continuing overproduction, which can be alleviated by expressing some milk. Many women leak milk when their breasts are stimulated during sexual activity. Wearing breast shells too long can also promote leaking. Cotton nursing pads tucked into your bra help minimize staining. Change pads frequently and avoid using plastic coverings, which can promote bacterial growth and skin problems. You can also stop the milk flow by pressing gently on your nipples.

PLUGGED OR CAKED MILK DUCT. A sore breast lump and decreased milk flow without a fever or other symptoms of mastitis (see below) may indicate an obstructed or plugged duct. Possible causes include infrequent nursing, incomplete softening or draining of the breast, and engorgement. To dislodge the plug, try applying a warm compress and then massaging the breast to stimulate milk flow just before breastfeeding. Breastfeed frequently on that side to clear the plugged area. If symptoms continue, see your physician.

MASTITIS. Mastitis is caused by a bacterial infection in the breast. It typically develops in only one breast and starts with fatigue, achy muscles, fever, and other flulike symptoms, followed by breast inflammation and pain. Mild cases may require only rest, frequent nursing (or pumping) to drain the breast, and warm compresses to relieve pain. More severe cases can be cleared up with antibiotics. Breastfeeding can and should continue in nearly all cases. If an abscess forms, it may have to be drained. See your doctor promptly if you develop symptoms or signs of mastitis.

Baby Problem Solving

Like most new mothers, Jasmine felt a bit overwhelmed by the responsibility of caring for a brand-new baby, even though her husband was supportive and both of them had prepared thoroughly at parenting classes. Four days after they brought their baby home, Jasmine was worried that she wasn't producing enough milk. Responding to her pediatrician's questions at an office visit, Jasmine told him that the baby nursed vigorously every 2 to 3 hours and slept after each feeding. Her breasts felt full before feedings and softened after the baby nursed. The baby had passed two loose stools each day since they came home, and Jasmine was changing wet diapers about six times a day.

"There's nothing to worry about," the pediatrician told Jasmine. "You're doing a great job and your baby is beautiful. Call me if you have any questions."

Wet diapers are an important guide to whether babies are feeding well. However, the absorbent qualities of some of the newest, stay-dry disposable diapers can make it hard to tell if a baby has urinated. It may be best to avoid super-absorbent diapers for the first few weeks, until you and your baby have settled into a routine.

SPITTING UP. Most babies spit up varying amounts of milk or formula, often for no apparent reason and with no health consequences. Spitting up, or reflux of stomach contents back into the esophagus, should not be confused with vomiting—the forceful expulsion of stomach contents. Reflux becomes a problem if the baby develops esophagitis, which causes pain. (In adults, this pain is called heartburn.) A baby with esophagitis becomes irritable shortly after feedings begin. The infant may appear hungry and start to feed eagerly, but then begin to cry or fuss

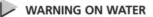

▷ WARNING ON WATER

Healthy infants do not need extra water. Breastmilk or formula provides all the fluids they need. A small amount of water may be needed in very hot weather, but check with your pediatrician on how much is safe. The American Academy of Pediatrics warns that during the exclusive nursing period (up to 6 months of age), giving a lot of water carries a risk of water intoxication and may interfere with breastmilk intake. With the introduction of solid foods, water can be added to your baby's diet.

as if in pain. If your baby has these symptoms or becomes fussy during feedings, consult your pediatrician. You probably don't need to worry about spitting up so long as your baby is growing normally, wetting at least six to eight diapers a day, and having normal bowel movements. To reduce spitting up, hold your baby quietly upright for a few minutes after each feeding. In bottle-fed infants, an intolerance to an ingredient in the formula or a response to supplements may trigger vomiting, but not spitting up. If you suspect a problem, consult your pediatrician. (Also see Chapter 7.)

GAS. When 2-week-old Alex cried hard after feedings, drew his knees up, and passed gas repeatedly, his mother called her pediatrician. "Is it colic? My mother warned me about it."

After a few questions, the pediatrician was able to reassure this anxious mother that her baby wasn't colicky. Alex was calmer after passing gas, he spat up very little, and he was sleeping well between feedings.

"Alex's digestive tract is getting used to food. It's developing a balance of the normal bacteria we need for digestion. The gas is a normal part of this process; it shows that your baby is adapting well to life on the outside."

COLIC. Dr. Stern's rule for recognizing colic: "You know your baby has colic when you have an irresistible urge to get him his own apartment." Colic is marked by periods of prolonged, inconsolable crying that seems to come from abdominal cramping and discomfort. The spells, which have no apparent cause, typically occur at about the same time every afternoon or evening. Colic usually develops between 2 and 6 weeks of age and disappears in 3 or 4 months. In contrast to simple gas, the crying does not stop after the baby passes gas. While colic lasts, both parents and baby go through acute suffering. No one knows what causes colic. It occurs more often in bottle-fed babies but can also appear in breastfed infants; it is also more common in first babies. Sometimes, but not very often, changing the mother's diet helps (see Chapter 15). You might try eliminating cow's milk from your diet as well as other sensitizing foods, such as wheat, peanuts, eggs, and seafood. You're more likely to be successful in calming your baby if you experiment with soothing tactics such as rocking, walking with him, playing music, or going for a car ride. You also should consult your pediatrician to make sure the crying is not due to a medical problem.

CONSTIPATION. Some breastfed babies go for several days without having a bowel movement. So long as the stool is soft and easily passed and your baby is growing normally, there's no need for c o n c e r n . B u t y o u should consult your pediatrician if the stools are hard or your baby's tummy is hard and distended.

DIARRHEA. Loose stools do not necessarily indicate diarrhea. If your baby has no other symptoms and is gaining normally, her runny stools may be what's normal for her. But if she has large, frequent, watery stools, a fever, or other symptoms, call your pediatrician. If your baby is dehydrated, a rehydrating solution may be needed. In most cases, breast- or bottle-feeding can continue until the problem clears up, but follow your pediatrician's instructions.

SLEEPY BABY. Most babies are born alert and are eager to feed in the first hour or so of life. Experts recommend feeding a newborn for about 30 minutes and to change breasts while she's still alert and interested. Typically, a baby will then fall asleep and wake up every 2 or 3 hours to nurse. But some babies are sleepy in the first day or two—they often need to be awakened to feed, and even then, they may fall asleep after only a few minutes of nursing. Often, cooling your baby down by removing some clothing or a blanket will help wake her up. Or try talking or singing to her, stroking her head, rubbing her buttocks or back, or wiping her face with a damp cloth. It's important that you get her to nurse for long enough to get the milk she needs for proper growth and also to drain your breasts to ensure steady milk production. If you have problems keeping her awake to feed, consult your pediatrician.

FUSSY EATER. Babies, like everyone else, have taste preferences. If your baby has been feeding normally and suddenly seems unhappy with your milk, suspect something you've eaten. The tastes of onions, garlic, cabbage, and other strong-flavored foods can pass into your milk, and the first time may surprise your baby. Most babies get to like new tastes; babies may even like the taste of garlic. If your baby stays fussy, try eliminating possibly offending foods, one at a time, for a week. Then try the eliminated food again. If it again provokes a reaction, eliminate the food until you stop nursing.

BREASTMILK JAUNDICE. The most common form of jaundice, called "physiologic jaundice of the newborn," affects two thirds of all babies and develops in the first few days after birth. Late-onset jaundice appears a little later or may be a continuation of the early jaundice. Your baby's skin may remain yellow for 6 to 12 weeks. The yellowing is caused by excess blood levels of bilirubin, a pigment normally eliminated by the liver. For unknown reasons, something in breast-milk triggers jaundice in susceptible babies. In nearly all cases, breastfeeding should continue, but your pediatrician will monitor your baby's bilirubin level. If the level is very high, you may be advised to stop breastfeeding for a day or so to lower the bilirubin level. During this time, you can keep up the milk flow with a breast pump until your baby is ready to breastfeed again.

WEAK SUCK. Most babies are born with a strong rooting reflex and have no trouble suckling, even when they are only minutes old. Occasionally, however, a baby has difficulty sucking. Telltale signs include losing hold of the breast, possible choking or gagging, and milk leaking from your baby's mouth. Sometimes a weak suck in a new-born is due to medications given to the mother during birth; if so, it should disappear as the medicines clear from your baby's system. Changing position to give your baby a better latch-on may help. But if the problem persists, your pediatrician should evaluate your baby for a possible physical problem or illness.

GROWTH. At about 6 months of age, babies who are exclusively breastfed may have a drop-off of weight in relation to length, which continues to increase normally. In fact, the baby's rate of growth may cross growth-chart percentiles. However, this is normal and no cause for concern so long as the length increases are steady.

TONGUE ABNORMALITIES. Rarely, a baby is born with a tongue abnormality that prevents proper latching on or suckling. Your pediatrician can advise you how to handle the problem.

CLEFT LIP. Babies born with a cleft lip can usually suckle normally, although the split in the lip will allow some milk to leak from your baby's mouth. You may have to experiment with positions to help your baby latch on; a nurse or lactation consultant can help you get started.

CLEFT PALATE. A cleft palate prevents a baby from effective suckling, but there are techniques to help babies feed. Also, a baby may be fitted with an appliance to temporarily seal the hole in the palate and make suckling easier. Breastmilk is particularly beneficial for infants with cleft palate because it reduces the risk of ear and lung infections, to which they are more susceptible.

Is Milk Really Enough?

Yes, for about 4 to 6 months of life. Pediatricians now agree that other foods should not be given until babies are about 6 months old. Still, many well-meaning grandparents, aunts, and others who reared their children in the 1960s and '70s advise earlier feeding of different foods.

When Gladys Evans became a mother in 1970, her obstetrician discouraged her from breastfeeding and her pediatrician respected her decision to use formula. Her baby, Sally, was healthy and active and, at her 8-week checkup, she had gained 3 pounds since birth. At that point, her pediatrician recommended starting Sally on rice cereal thinned with formula and progressing to puréed and strained fruit a week or so later, followed by strained vegetables a couple of weeks after that.

"At first, Sally simply spit out most of the cereal," Gladys recalls, "but then I tried putting the food way back on her tongue so she had to swallow it. After that, I didn't have any problems getting her to eat."

Now that Gladys is a grandmother, it's understandable that she is worried about the way Sally is feeding her own baby. "He's almost 5 months old and he's still on nothing but breastmilk," Gladys explains. "Is this really enough?"

Changing Views

As this typical case illustrates, views on infant feeding have changed over the last few decades. Pediatricians and nutrition experts now know that giving foods other than breastmilk or formula in the first few months of life is detrimental for several reasons:

- Until babies are at least 4 months old, their digestive systems have trouble breaking down the starches and components of other foods.
- An immature digestive system may allow whole

 COMMON MYTHS ABOUT BREASTFEEDING

Myth	Facts
You can't get pregnant while breastfeeding.	While it's true that breastfeeding prevents ovulation in some women, it is not a reliable form of birth control. Talk to your doctor about an acceptable form of contraception. Avoid estrogen-containing birth-control pills.
You need to "toughen" your nipples before your baby is born.	Normal nipples need no advance preparation or "toughening." Flat or inverted nipples, however, may be helped by certain exercises (see Inverted or Flat Nipples, p. 13).
Small breasts don't produce as much milk as large ones	Breast size has nothing to do with the amount of milk they produce.
Breastfeeding will ruin the shape of your breasts	Most women find that their breasts go back to their pre-pregnancy size and shape after they stop nursing. Age and weight gain have more effect on breast size than nursing.
Sexual arousal while breastfeeding is abnormal.	Many women experience sexual arousal while nursing. Breast stimulation is an important aspect of sexual activity, so it stands to reason that nursing can also arouse sexual feelings. In addition, oxytocin—the hormone released during breastfeeding—is also released during orgasm, another reason why nursing can be sexually stimulating.
All babies should be weaned before their first birthday.	When to stop breastfeeding is a highly personal decision and varies considerably according to custom and individual preferences. Some women stop breastfeeding after a few months; others are still nursing when their children are age 3 or even older. It's all a matter of what's right for you and your child.

proteins to be absorbed, thus setting the stage for an allergic reaction, especially if there is a family history of allergies. By 4 months, the digestive system can break down proteins into their amino acid building blocks, which are less likely to provoke allergies.

■ When a spoon touches a young baby's tongue, it triggers an automatic extrusion reflex, in which the tongue thrusts forward and prevents swallowing. This reflex disappears at about 3 to 4 months of age.

Breastmilk provides all the nutrients that a healthy baby needs for about the first 6 months of life. Breastfeeding also benefits the mother (see The Special Health Benefits of Breastfeeding, p. 9).

Eating for Two

During pregnancy and while breastfeeding, you are eating for both yourself and your baby. Indeed, your health and nutrition during pregnancy are big factors in determining your baby's nutritional needs. Ideally, sound infant nutrition begins even before conception. It's a good idea to have a thorough pre-pregnancy checkup to make sure you're not anemic or don't have hidden nutritional, metabolic, or other problems. Your doctor will advise you about what supplements you need during pregnancy and how much weight you should gain, as well as foods and substances you should avoid. Be sure to tell your doctor if you follow a vegetarian diet or one that excludes certain foods. It may be advisable for you to take a vitamin supplement during pregnancy and while breastfeeding.

As part of your plan to breastfeed, you should continue eating a healthful diet that provides the extra energy and nutrients you need to make milk. In the past, breastfeeding mothers were advised to consume an extra 400 or 500 calories a day and to drink at least eight glasses of water and other fluids. Doctors now recognize that there are no set rules—some women may need an extra 500 calories, while others will gain unwanted pounds by eating this much. The best rule is to eat and drink enough to satisfy your hunger and thirst. Follow the Food Guide Pyramid (see p. 90), with ample fresh or lightly processed fruits and vegetables to provide essential vitamins and minerals. Nursing mothers eating a balanced diet do not require any added calcium. If there is a family history of allergies, they may prefer to minimize cow's milk consumption while nursing so that their babies are not exposed to excess cow's milk protein.

Certain strongly flavored foods and spices can affect the taste and composition of breastmilk and may cause digestive problems in babies. A common culprit is cabbage. Most babies develop a liking for garlic and onions after the initial surprise. Garlic and spices need not be avoided unless your baby continues to react negatively to them. Excessive caffeine (more than five cups a day of coffee or other caffeinated beverages, such as tea and sodas) may make your baby jittery and fussy. In addition, both caffeine and nicotine decrease milk flow. If something in your diet seems to upset your baby's appetite or disposition, eliminate it for the time being. You may, however, need to keep a food diary to identify the offending food.

Important No-Nos

Because much of what you eat and drink can enter your breastmilk, it's important that you avoid any substance that can harm your baby. Here are a few commonsense rules to follow:

Always check with your pediatrician before taking any medication, both prescription and over-the-counter products, as well as herbal or natural remedies. Prescription drugs that are contraindicated during breastfeeding include some blood-pressure-lowering medications, certain antibiotics, antithyroid medications, and cancer chemotherapy drugs. Many people mistakenly assume that over-the-counter drugs and herbal remedies have no adverse effects; this is not true. Even aspirin in breastmilk can cause problems in a baby. Herbal remedies can be toxic, especially to babies. However, most over-the-counter products sold to relieve common symptoms such as headache and indigestion are acceptable, though you should check with your doctor before taking them.

IF YOU SMOKE, NOW IS THE TIME TO STOP. Not only does nicotine enter your breastmilk, but it also lowers the amount of milk you produce. If you can't quit, at least cut down as much as you can and never smoke in the hour or so before nursing. Remember, too, that secondhand smoke is especially dangerous for your baby. Don't allow smoking in your house or car and certainly not in the presence of your baby.

AVOID ALCOHOL WHILE YOU ARE BREASTFEEDING. Doctors agree that substance abusers (those who use drugs such as marijuana, cocaine, heroin, and amphetamines) should not nurse at all. Alcohol and these other substances pass into breastmilk and are harmful to your baby.

AVOID ENVIRONMENTAL TOXINS AS MUCH AS POSSIBLE. In some areas, breastfeeding mothers are advised not to eat freshwater fish because they may contain PCBs, potent cancer-causing chemicals. Pesticides can also enter breastmilk; always wash fresh fruits and vegetables before eating them.

ISSUES PARENTS OFTEN RAISE ABOUT BREASTFEEDING

I'm afraid of what's going to happen once I take my baby home from the hospital. What if I'm having problems breastfeeding and my baby isn't getting enough to eat?
If you have concerns after you leave the hospital, call your physician or your baby's pediatrician. He or she will be able to answer your questions and may suggest the help of a lactation consultant . Many of these counselors make home visits. Your doctor may also refer you to a support group for nursing mothers. (See p. 6 for more about breastfeeding instruction.)

How will I know when my baby is ready to start breastfeeding?
Like all other baby mammals, newborn humans are almost always alert and eager to suckle shortly after their birth. Provided there are no problems, your baby may be put to the breast immediately after birth. You'll soon learn the cry that tells you she's hungry! (Read about getting started with breastfeeding on p. 6.)

Does breastfeeding make a difference to children's health in the long term?
Breastfed babies have fewer allergies, intestinal upsets, ear infections, and

other common childhood illnesses than formula-fed infants. Not only that, but children who were breastfed as babies have lower rates of diabetes, asthma, and other chronic disorders long after infancy. (For more about the health benefits of breastfeeding, see p. 9.)

I hoped to breastfeed my baby but my doctor says I shouldn't because I have to take medication for a chronic condition. Does this mean it'll be harder for me to bond with my child?
Your doctor is advising you to do what's best for both you and your baby. Like millions of other parents you'll find bot-tle-feeding a warm, loving, and fulfilling experience. Cuddle your baby, gaze into her eyes, and coo and talk to her as you feed her. This is all part of bonding. (Read more about bottle-feeding techniques on p. 10.)

If my baby doesn't finish a bottle of formula, how long is it safe to keep the leftovers?
Never keep leftover formula or breastmilk. Germs and enzymes from your baby's mouth normally enter the bottle and can spoil the formula. Use a fresh bottle for every feeding. (Read about how to sterilize and clean bottles and nipples on p. 12.)

CHAPTER 2

Expanding Your Baby's Diet

After a rocky start, Maria and Jose Lopez eased into the breastfeeding routines of their infant Ricky and developed confidence in their abilities to know when he was hungry and how long he should nurse.

"I thought I had a system that worked," says Maria. "But when it came time to introduce solid foods, I didn't have a clue." And she found advice from friends and family more confusing than helpful.

"Everyone had different advice to offer, about everything from when I should start offering solid foods to Ricky, to how much I should expect him to eat—even what those first foods should be."

Shifting Views

Not only does personal advice vary, professional advice has shifted over time. Before 1920, solid or supplemental foods were seldom recommended for infants until one year of age. Then, in the 1950s, the tables turned and the trend was to introduce supplemental foods as early as possible—some even advocated within the first few days of life. Today, the American Academy of Pediatrics recommends that parents introduce the first supplemental foods somewhere between 4 and 6 months of age. A child's readiness depends on his developmental level. Whereas one child may be ready both mentally and physically to take on new foods at 4 months of age, another may be barely ready to

Most infants make the transition from all breastmilk or formula to eating other foods at about 4 to 6 months. Whenever it's practical, the whole family should eat together. This helps your baby develop an eating pattern that lets him interact with other family members at mealtime.

take on the task at 6 months. Yet both children are in the "normal" range of development. If you wait much longer than 6 months, however, your child may be less willing to accept solid foods. Even after the introduction of solid foods, breastfeeding can and should continue.

How to Know If the Time Is Right

It's easy to worry that you may be putting your child at risk of overeating if you introduce other foods too soon, or that he's developmentally delayed if he's not ready until much later. Such fears can be made worse by well-meaning advice from friends and family members. Though advice from those more experienced than you can sometimes be helpful, the best advice is to know your own child, so you'll be better able to recognize clues that he's ready for you to introduce him to supplemental foods. Don't be in a rush. Some infants like to take their own sweet time accepting new foods, and forcing the issue will only make the transition more stressful for you and your baby. Above all, relax and allow your growing infant to experiment and develop her own eating patterns and rituals that become both familiar and comforting—in short, something she looks forward to.

By 3 to 4 months of age, the child loses the "extrusion reflex," which makes an infant instinctively push his tongue out when anything other than liquid is placed in his mouth. You can expect that by 5 to 6 months of age, most children will be able to express their desire for food. For example, until recently you've probably been able to eat your own food without attracting much attention from your child. But now, he's likely to show more than a passing interest in what's on your plate, leaning forward, drooling, and even opening his mouth. Your child may also cry more often between feedings, a signal that breastmilk or formula alone isn't enough. Waiting until your child is ready before introducing solid food makes the process easier on everyone. Not only will he accept solid food more readily in the beginning, but it may also make the transition to family foods easier and shorter.

Step by Step, but Not Set in Stone

It's not always a smooth transition from your child's first taste of supplemental food to the time he's eating the same food as the rest of the family.

Your infant has a mind of his own and may have strong opinions about what you're trying to get him to eat. While some children enthusiastically embrace the idea of solid food, almost as if to say, "What took you so long?" with others it may take weeks of gentle prodding with a loaded spoon before they'll venture into unfamiliar territory. Once you've decided that both you and your baby are ready for the feeding challenge, keep these three basic points in mind.

1. FEED SIMPLE, BASIC FOODS FIRST. Rice cereal is most often recommended, because it is gluten-free and less often associated with an allergic response. (Gluten is a protein that can sometimes trigger allergic reactions.) However, in rare instances, a child may even be sensitive to rice cereal. The cereal can be mixed with breastmilk or warm formula (later on, fruit juice is another option) and made either thick or thin, depending on your child's eating skills. But in general, use about 1 teaspoon of cereal mixed with 4 to 5 tea-

▷ **THE FIRST SOLID FOODS ARE SEMILIQUIDS**

Solid foods for babies are not really solid at all. The first solid food is usually semiliquid ground rice cereal. Once your child has mastered that, she can move up to strained or mashed foods and, somewhere between 7 and 10 months, finely chopped table foods. (At this stage, all foods should be milled, or otherwise have a texture that readily dissolves in the mouth. Foods that need to be chewed are likely to cause choking until the child has both the teeth and the muscular coordination to deal with them.) The transition is a gradual process that varies greatly from one baby to another. If your baby was a preemie, you may find the transition particularly slow and difficult. Some children have an especially hard time adjusting to the new textures of foods and may cough, gag, or even vomit when you try to introduce new foods. If that's the case, you'll need to introduce foods much more slowly, making the addition of solid foods a longer-than-usual process. But eventually, even children with such extreme oral sensitivity come around and are ready and willing to eat when it's time for a meal.

If your chief reason for introducing solid food is to get your night owl of a child to sleep through the night, think again, because it won't work. Despite the widespread belief that just a bit of rice cereal will do the trick, research doesn't back it up. Your baby will be able to sleep for extended periods only when he has reached the right level of developmental maturity and he is capable of comforting himself when awake and not hungry.

spoons of breastmilk, formula, or warm water. Around 6 months of age, your baby's natural iron stores are depleted. The extra iron in infant cereals provides about 30 percent to 45 percent of your baby's daily requirement for iron. Iron from cereal is well absorbed and should bring your baby's iron stores back to where they need to be. Infant cereals also provide significant amounts of thiamin, riboflavin, niacin, calcium, vitamin B_6, and phosphorus. While there are also high-protein infant cereals to choose from, a healthy infant who is growing normally has no need for the extra protein they provide. A single-grain, iron-fortified infant cereal is the best choice.

2. GIVE YOUR INFANT SMALL SERVINGS. If the 1 or 2 teaspoons he eats seem like a minuscule amount, don't worry. It's fine for his first few times. You don't want him to eat so much solid food that it replaces the breastmilk he needs. At this point, solid food is merely an addition to his breastmilk-based diet. Even an experienced 6-month-old infant may eat only about 3 to 4 tablespoons at a meal. The rest of his nutrient needs will be met by breastmilk and formula, at least for a while. Your baby's calorie needs vary depending on how fast he is growing and how active he is. Infants aged 6 months to 1 year need about 50 calories per pound, for a total of about 850 calories a day from both solids and breastmilk or formula. It's important to remember,

however, that babies don't eat calories; they eat food, and they regulate their energy intake according to their needs.

3. LIMIT NEW FOODS TO ONE AT A TIME. Apart from its being a little overwhelming to your child, if you offer something new at every meal, it becomes difficult to identify adverse reactions to specific foods, should they occur. Your baby has plenty of time to experiment with new tastes and textures. One-at-a-time is the best approach for now, and only one new food every 2 or 3 days.

Though certain foods are more likely to cause problems, any food has the potential to trigger either a food allergy or a food intolerance. Children are most likely to have adverse reactions to food in their first year; the risk is much lower after age 3. The younger your child is when you introduce supplemental food, the greater the risk that he'll have an allergic reaction. And if you or other family members suffer from food allergies,

▶ A NEW ROLE FOR DAD

If you're a nursing mom, adding solid foods gives Dad the chance, at last, to participate in feeding his baby. Encourage him to share in your infant's discovery of new foods.

Don't let well-intentioned advice lead you astray. One common piece of advice says if you can't get your child to accept solid food readily, then you should put a little watered-down rice cereal in a bottle with some breastmilk or formula. Widen the hole in the nipple, they say, and you've got a no-fuss way to give your child solid food. But this teaches the infant nothing about the mechanics or social aspects of eating solid foods. Also, it risks overloading your child with calories.

the chances are greater that your child will, too. But true food allergies, which set the immune system into action, are rare. It's more likely that your child will experience an intolerance to a particular food or ingredient. A food intolerance can cause diarrhea, bloating, and gas, and is often mistaken for a food allergy, but, unlike food allergies, it does not involve the immune system. Among the foods best avoided until about one year of age, because they are most likely to cause problems, are wheat, egg whites, citrus fruits and juices, and cow's milk. Check ingredient labels carefully. Some high-protein and mixed-grain cereals contain wheat, though you won't always be able to tell by looking at the cereal name on the front label.

If your child appears to have a reaction to a particular food, remove it from her diet for 1 to 3 months before offering it again. The basic rule here is, if at first you don't succeed, try again later. If the food provokes a reaction on a subsequent try, eliminate it for several months. Research sug-gests that by one year of age, most babies are able to tolerate foods that had earlier caused a reaction.

Symptoms such as diarrhea, skin rashes, wheezing, nausea and vomiting, cramps, headache, or hives in the absence of fever suggest a true food allergy. (For more information on food allergies and food sensitivities, see Chapter 15.)

When Your Infant Says "When"

Ramiel, at 6 months, took to cereals, fruits, and strained carrots like a duckling to water. But when his mother, Naïma, offered him strained broccoli, Ramiel screwed up his face, gagged, squawked, and spat it out. Naïma went back to the tried-and-true for the next few meals, then mixed a little broccoli purée with Ramiel's favorite strained carrots. After a couple of successful mixed feedings, Naïma again served strained broccoli. This time, Ramiel devoured the vegetable. Naïma realized that Ramiel's facial expressions didn't mean he disliked the food; it was just new and different, and he needed to get used to it gradually.

You may get some mixed signals about whether your child likes what you're feeding him. Sweet foods, like applesauce, are usually accepted with a

▷ **START THE MEAL WITH SOLIDS**

Save the bottle until your baby has finished eating the solids. She'll be hungriest at the start of the meal, and more willing to try new foods. Remember, in the beginning, solid foods are an addition to—not a replacement for—breastmilk or formula.

Though what to feed your child is the major issue, where to feed her can sometimes be just as perplexing. If your child is sitting up, then it's time to bring out the high chair. However, if she's ready to eat but has not yet mastered the skill of sitting upright and unsupported for any length of time, then you'll need to pick a spot that's comfortable for both of you. You may find it works just fine if she sits in your lap (put all breakables out of reach), or you might try an infant carrier or motionless swing. She may be slightly reclined, but she should be upright enough to eat and swallow without choking. Whatever eating spot you choose, remember it's for a very short time. As soon as she's able to sit on her own, a high chair at the family dinner table is the best feeding spot. And be sure to use the chair's safety straps at all times.

look of satisfaction. But a puckered-up face in response to a new vegetable isn't necessarily a sign that he doesn't want more. It may just be a reaction to a new and unexpected taste or texture. Offer it again—if he opens his mouth, he wants more, despite what his facial contortions may suggest. If it's still a no-go, give it a rest and try again a few days later. Parents often unconsciously give signals for liking or disliking foods, especially when they try to feed children foods they themselves don't like. Try not to let your expression influence your child when serving a food you don't enjoy.

Don't be surprised if your infant's reaction to his first solid food is to push it out with his tongue and dribble most of it down his chin. It's normal. Remember, he's never had anything thicker than breastmilk or formula before, and this may take some getting used to. Try diluting it more for the first few times, then gradually thicken the texture.

Eventually you'll learn your child's signals that he's had enough: He may lean back, close his mouth tight, or turn his head. When his eye-to-hand coordination improves, he may even try to knock the spoon out of your hand. That's your

signal to stop feeding. Don't expect him to have the same appetite at every meal. The appetite of any healthy baby will vary. Sometimes he'll surprise you at just how much food he can hold, while other times he'll leave you frustrated over his lack of interest in food.

There are no hard and fast rules about when to introduce new foods to your baby's diet, but the chart on page 28 offers some basic guidelines. Notice that the time frames overlap to allow for the wide range of developmental stages among babies of the same age.

When Your Baby Can Feed Himself

For Trudi, the first few weeks of baby Hannelore's life were a delight. Hannelore fed well, slept when she wasn't feeding, and looked like a porcelain doll tucked tightly in her bassinet. However, when Hannelore began to show a more demanding personality, Trudi found the baby trying. As Hannelore grew used to solid foods, she would reach for the spoon or plunge her hands into her bowl, if Trudi left it within reach. A fastidious housekeeper, Trudi would interrupt the meal to wash the baby and change her clothes. By the

4 to 8 months	Begin iron-fortified rice cereal.
6 to 8 months	Introduce fruits, other cereals, vegetables, and diluted noncitrus juices.
7 to 10 months	Offer strained or mashed fruits and vegetables like bananas or applesauce, egg yolk, and some textured table foods (in no particular order); finely cut and chopped meat or poultry.
9 to 12 months	Introduce soft combination foods such as casseroles, macaroni and cheese, and spaghetti; yogurt, cheese; beans.
After 12 months	Give whole cow's milk.

time they resumed the meal, Hannelore was screaming, hungry, but too upset to eat, while Trudi was angry with the baby not only for making a mess but also for refusing the food that she had prepared. One day Trudi screamed at the baby, "I have better things to do than feed you and clean up after you all day long!"

Noting Trudi's tension and Hannelore's fretfulness at the next checkup, their pediatrician carefully probed until he got to the root of the problem. He sympathized with Trudi; it is difficult, he agreed, to put up with messes and disruptions when you are used to a calm, orderly routine. But he also pointed out that Hannelore was quite advanced for a baby not quite one year old, and she shouldn't be expected to act like a big girl for a long time yet.

The doctor explained that the sooner Hannelore was allowed to make a little mess, the sooner she'd learn to be clean, but it wouldn't happen overnight. He suggested that Trudi feed Hannelore in the kitchen instead of the dining room, and spread newspapers or a sheet of plastic under the high chair to catch the mess. He urged her to give Hannelore finger foods, as well as a spoon and unbreakable bowl, so she could learn to feed herself, as she longed to do. If Trudi found

herself getting tense and angry, perhaps her husband would give the baby her evening meal, or Trudi could ask a friend or neighbor to sit with her and help feed the baby during Hannelore's midday meal.

Somewhere around 7 months to 9 months of age, infants learn to put objects in their mouths and, given the opportunity, will try to feed themselves. Once your child has a well-developed pincer grasp and can pick up objects between his thumb and forefinger, any food he can pick up and bring to his mouth can be considered a "finger food." Foods that dissolve easily—like baby crackers, pieces of bread, plain cookies, sliced cheese, finger sandwiches, and dry cereals—are good first choices. This is also a good time to let your baby gradually get used to handling a spoon. You can let him play with a spare while you do the feeding. And when he finally decides to go it alone, be prepared for cleaning up to take almost as long as the meal itself.

About this same time, you may want to try allowing your infant to take a few sips from a cup with your help. Many breastfed babies never use a bottle and, instead, move directly to the cup. A two-handled plastic "sippy" cup is a good

BABY'S DIET PLAN

By the end of the transition from all breastmilk or formula to regular food with breastmilk or formula or regular milk (typically between 12 and 18 months), your child's minimum daily intake should look something like this:

Food	Servings
Whole milk	16 to 24 ounces
Fruits and vegetables	4 to 8 tablespoons
Breads and cereals	4 servings (a serving equals $1/4$ slice of bread or 2 tablespoons of rice, potatoes, pasta, etc.)
Meat, poultry, fish, eggs	2 servings of about $1/2$ ounce or 1 tablespoon each

first choice, though until your child is about 10 to 12 months old, more liquid may end up on her and the floor than in her mouth. Still, it's important to remember that play and experimentation are part of your child's mealtime, and are essential to her growing independence. Follow her lead and tune in to clues that she's still hungry or that mealtime is over. If you try to force-feed her, she may throw her food or "pouch" it, holding it in her cheeks without swallowing. Prodding her to eat more when she's had enough also can cause gagging. But above all, remember never to leave your child alone and unattended at mealtime. She doesn't know her own limitations and could easily choke from eating too fast or stuffing too much food in her mouth at one time. And if you have older children in the house, make sure that they don't try to feed your infant what they're eating.

When you make the switch from breastmilk or formula to regular milk after one year, don't be tempted to give your child fat-free, low-fat, or even reduced-fat milk. Although a lower-fat milk is the best choice for children after age 2 and for adults, your baby needs the fat calories whole

milk offers. You shouldn't consider lower-fat milk an option until after your child's second birthday.

Grocery Shopping for Your Baby

One of the first decisions you'll have to make before you mark the calendar for your baby's first "solid" meal is whether to make it yourself or buy prepared

 SENSITIVE MOUTHS AND COARSER TEXTURES

Some babies find it hard to get used to coarser textures, especially if they come across a lump in a "smooth" food. A typical offender is a lump or strand of fruit pulp in yogurt. These children may have unusually sensitive mouths; some are also oversensitive to loud sounds and bright lights. Be patient and work on intoducing new sensations gradually. Try to make sure that familiar foods don't hide unwelcome surprises. In time, your sensitive eater will accept a wide variety of textures.

baby food in jars. There is no "correct" answer. It depends on your budget, your lifestyle, and your concerns. Here are your main choices.

HOME-MADE FOODS. One advantage to preparing your baby's food is that it gets him used to what your family normally eats, instead of a jar of some commercial combination that you would never serve your family. Cooking and mashing simple foods like carrots, potatoes, squash, and bananas is easy. But preparation may require a little forethought and time as your child's taste horizons and eating skills expand to include foods such as peas, corn, green beans, peaches, and pineapple, which must be puréed or blended to transform them to textures your child can handle with ease. A hand-turned food mill with disks for different textures is inexpensive and easy to use.

For healthful nutrition, bake, broil, or steam foods. When boiling vegetables, use very little water, to preserve nutrients. Try to cook fresh vegetables within a day after you buy them. Vitamin C and several B vitamins can be lost while fresh produce sits in the vegetable bin in your refrigerator. If you're using the same foods as the rest of the family, separate your baby's portion before adding salt. And when buying canned or frozen foods, avoid those with salt, sugar, or added fat. If time is of the essence and convenience is top priority in your household, then making it yourself may not always be the best option. Some parents prefer to make baby foods for home use and keep a stock of commercial jars for traveling and emergencies. If you make foods yourself, be sure to take food safety precautions (see p. 32) when handling and preparing your baby's food.

COMMERCIAL FOODS. Ready-to-eat baby food in jars is convenient. There's no fuss, it's portable, and the foods come in a wide variety of flavors and ingredients. Baby foods today range from simple strained fruits to exotic tropical fruit dessert and organic lentils and rice dinner. You won't have to worry about the sodium content because salt is no longer added to commercially prepared baby foods. Some dinners and desserts do, however, have added sugar or modified food starch. While

▷ **PREPARING PORTIONS**

Remove and warm as much food as you think your baby will want to eat at a meal. If you prepare too much, throw out the leftovers. If you put leftovers back in the jar, it's an invitation for bacteria to grow, and any enzymes from baby's saliva will thin out the food.

Warm baby foods only to body temperature. If you're using the microwave, remove the container's cover and heat for only a few seconds at reduced power, being careful not to overheat. Microwaving can create "hot spots" in the food that can burn your child's mouth. Moreover, thick foods like strained meats and egg yolk, if warmed while still in the jar, can easily overheat in the microwave and can splatter or explode. To be safe, remove the food from the jar and place it in a microwave-safe dish—or don't warm it in the microwave at all.

both ingredients are safe, they take the place of more nutritious ingredients. Most baby food manufacturers categorize their products according to age-appropriate stages, usually stages 1, 2, 3, and toddler foods—finely puréed foods for first-timers and thicker and more textured foods for older babies. But, instead of making your choice more simple, it can sometimes be confusing, since manufacturers don't use standardized ages and stages. Two rules apply across the board: Begin with stage 1 foods for beginners, and don't offer your child toddler foods, which often contain chunks, until he is an experienced eater.

Until now your baby has required little or no fluids in addition to breastmilk or formula. But now that solid foods are becoming a regular part of his diet, so should additional fluids. Water is the best choice for quenching thirst without adding extra calories, particularly in hot weather. Be sure to offer water at feeding time so that your infant gets all the fluid he needs.

ORGANIC FOODS. Organic baby foods, available in some supermarkets and health food stores, have grown in popularity as people have become increasingly concerned about the effects of pesticides and other agricultural chemicals on children's health. Organic crops are grown in soil fertilized with manure and compost instead of synthetic chemicals. Organically produced foods, including meats, are from sources free of added hormones, antibiotics, dyes, waxes, and other additives. (Also see Chapter 13.)

While some parents are concerned that children's exposure to pesticides, especially from fruits and vegetables, may be great relative to their size, the levels of pesticides found in produce are typically well below the safety levels set by the Environmental Protection Agency. Moreover, the processing involved in making baby food reduces

▷ **NO HONEY FOR BABIES**

Although honey may seem like a healthy food to feed your infant, don't do it. Honey has been associated with infant botulism, an illness that can be fatal. The American Academy of Pediatrics recommends that honey not be given to infants younger than 12 months. That's because spores of *Clostridium botulinum* can sometimes grow and produce toxins in the infant's intestinal tract, causing a potentially fatal illness. An adult's intestinal tract has the ability to prevent the growth of the clostridium spores.

pesticide residues to such a degree that the final product has no detectable residues left. Experts warn that the risks of not including fruits and vegetables in children's diets are far greater than any potential risk from pesticides at the levels currently allowed.

Should you feed your baby organic foods? That's a decision only you can make based on your lifestyle and your pocketbook, since commercial organic baby food—or organic produce for making baby foods at home—generally costs considerably more than the standard brands.

Tips for Using Commercial Baby Food

- Check the "use by" date on the container to make sure the date hasn't passed.
- Store unopened jars in your kitchen cabinet at room temperature.
- Make sure the vacuum seal button on the lid is down. If it has popped up, discard the jar.
- When you open a jar, listen for a "whoosh"

"pop" sound. If the center of the lid pops up, that's your sign that the seal is good and the food is safe for your baby.

- Remove as much food from the jar as you think your baby will eat. Never feed from the jar.
- Once a jar has been opened, refrigerate the unused portion of the jar immediately. Leftovers should stay fresh for 1 to 2 days.
- Most manufacturers warn against freezing regular baby food. Though it is safe to do, it changes the texture. (Some manufacturers offer lines of frozen baby foods that are specially prepared to preserve texture and flavor.)

Food Safety Tips for Your Baby's Meals

- Keep tools and work spaces as clean as possible. Cutting boards, sponges, and dishrags are notorious breeding grounds for bacteria that can cause foodborne illnesses.
- Wash hands thoroughly with hot, soapy water before preparation and in between handling raw and cooked foods. Use disposable paper towels or freshly laundered, dry cloths.
- Cook meat to a temperature of at least 160°F (the United States Department of Agriculture recommends using an instant-read meat thermometer for the preparation of all meat, since meat can appear done at lower temperatures).
- Don't store cooked food for more than 2 days.

Whether you make your own baby foods or buy regular or organic commercial foods, the same basics apply. Here are some specific examples of foods to help you follow the general timeline suggested in Making the Transition, p. 28.

CEREALS. Start off with plain rice cereal. After the high-risk allergy period has passed, add barley or oatmeal cereals, trying one at a time to start. After 6 months, you may want to try a cereal and fruit combination. You can buy ready-made combinations such as rice and bananas or prunes and oatmeal, or you can mix your own. The thickness and texture should depend on your child's eating skills.

In the beginning, your infant is likely to eat only a few teaspoons, but eventually he should be eating about $1/2$ cup of iron-fortified cereal a day. If no other iron source is provided, it's recommended that an iron-fortified cereal be a part of your child's diet until about 18 months of age. If,

 WHOLE-WHEAT VS. WHEAT: WHAT'S THE DIFFERENCE?

Whole-wheat bread offers a nutritional advantage over white bread, which is also marketed as "wheat" bread. Both are made from wheat flour; the key is to know the difference. Whole-wheat bread contains the fiber-rich outer bran layer and the nutritious inner germ of the wheat kernel, which delivers vitamins B_6 and E, folic acid, copper, magnesium, manganese, and zinc. By contrast, in wheat bread made from refined wheat flour, the bran and germ are eliminated. Both whole-wheat bread and wheat bread are fortified with niacin, thiamin, iron, and folic acid. You need to read labels carefully to make the right choice. Don't be misled by the terms "wheat," "made with whole wheat," "unbleached wheat," or even "multi-grain." Instead, look for 100 percent whole wheat as the first ingredient listed.

Don't be alarmed if you notice a change in the color and odor of your infant's bowel movements after he starts eating solid food. Vegetables such as beets, carrots, spinach, and peas are especially likely to cause changes in color. Yellow, green, or red bowel movements are not unusual. What your baby eats can also affect the texture and consistency of his bowel movements. Banana stools come out looking like tiny worms, pear stools like small stones. If, however, your baby has a lot of gas, diarrhea, or stomach upset after eating a specific food, stop feeding it for a few weeks, then try again.

however, your child is also drinking an iron-fortified formula, taking a multivitamin with iron, and has begun eating meat, he may be getting too much iron. Talk to your pediatrician to be sure you're giving your child the right combination of iron-containing foods and supplements.

BREADS. When you introduce your infant to breads and cereals, you're also introducing him for the first time to wheat, a potential allergen. If he's about 6 to 8 months of age, it's probably okay. But if anyone in your family has been diagnosed with a food allergy, there is an increased chance that your child, too, may be allergic. If you want to offer wheat-free breads and cereals, try rice crackers or corn or rice cereals. Read labels carefully. Wheat may be a "hidden" ingredient. If wheat is not a problem, offer small pieces of whole-wheat bread, pita bread, or bagels. Unsweetened cereals are good finger snacks.

FRUITS. All ready-to-eat baby fruits in jars are fortified with vitamin C and provide about 35 percent to 45 percent of your baby's vitamin C needs per serving. If you choose commercial varieties, start off with single-ingredient fruits before progressing to two- or three-fruit combinations and then fruits with added tapioca or rice. Soft, easy-to-mash fruits canned in juice, water, or light syrup usually work well. If you go with regular canned fruits, be sure to include a good source of vitamin C such as vitamin C–fortified juice in your child's daily diet. Fresh fruits like peaches, pears, plums, or bananas can be mashed, diced, or cut into chunks, depending on your child's level of skill. If your baby is already eating vegetables and meat, serve them first at lunch or dinner. Children love the sweet taste of fruit and, given the choice, may pick fruit over other foods.

JUICES. Fruit juices, such as orange, apple, and pear, tend to become favorites, sometimes to the exclusion of other foods. While they are moderately nutritious—all baby juices are fortified with vitamin C—it's easy to let your child go overboard.

Don't make the common mistake of offering unlimited access to fruit juice. Not only does it dampen your child's appetite at mealtime, but drinking too much juice can also cause cramping and diarrhea (also see Chapter 7). Research suggests that pear juice is the worst offender, followed by apple and grape juices, which are the most common ingredients in infant juice mixtures. If you frequently offer your child juice, dilute it half-and-half with water. Limit servings to no more than 4 ounces ($^1/_2$ cup).

There's a wide variety of juices made specifi-

This is a time of rapid transition for your baby. Don't expect to keep to any particular feeding routine for very long. The one thing you can count on during this time is change. Let your infant set the pace. Follow her cues as to what she's ready to try, and you'll have fewer feeding problems.

cally for infants and toddlers. While they are conveniently packaged, they are considerably more expensive than regular frozen or bottled juices. You can do just as well buying an "adult" juice fortified with vitamin C, but avoid unpasteurized ciders and juices because they may contain harmful bacteria (see Chapter 13). You can also try offering your child low-sodium vegetable juices. Though not appealing to every infant's taste buds, they are nutritious additions to the diet. Steer clear of regular bottled or canned vegetable juices, however, which are often quite high in sodium. Of course, water is always a good choice for quenching your child's thirst.

VEGETABLES. If you make your own baby foods, be aware that home-prepared spinach, beets, turnips, and collard greens are not good choices during early infancy. They may contain enough nitrates to interfere with the transport of hemoglobin through the blood. Commercially prepared vegetables are safe because the manufacturers test for nitrates. Peas, corn, green beans, squash, mixed vegetables, and sweet potatoes are better choices for home-made baby foods.

MEATS. Somewhere between 7 and 10 months of age, your baby will probably be eating three meals a day, and as solid food begins to make up more of his intake, breastmilk or formula intake decreases. That's when it becomes important to feed him protein from other sources, such as ground or very finely chopped meat or poultry.

You may also find out that meat is generally at the bottom of the list of your baby's favorite foods. Acceptance may take longer than for other foods. It probably will be better accepted if it's puréed, warmed slightly, and mixed with a favorite vegetable. (At this age, infants still tend to gag, and do not have molars for chewing. Even finely chopped meats may be hard to handle and cause choking.) If your child is not getting another good source of iron, it's important that he have some iron-rich meat in his diet, although he doesn't need meat every day. A $2^1/2$-ounce jar of a commercially prepared, age-appropriate meat dish provides about 50 percent of an infant's recommended daily protein allowance. It also provides significant amounts of riboflavin, niacin, and vitamin B_6, as well as iron. Though in the past egg yolks were recommended as a good source of iron, the iron they contain is not easily absorbed. Iron-fortified cereals and meat are the best iron sources for your infant.

MIXED FOODS. Last on the list of additions to your baby's diet, mixed foods can range from tuna casseroles and macaroni and cheese to toddler "dinners" in jars and frozen entrées. The so-called infant dinners in jars are more appropriate as vegetable servings than as meat servings. That's because most contain small amounts of meat and some vegetables along with starch fillers and seasonings. The ingredients in these dinners vary widely, so read ingredient labels carefully if your child has a food allergy or food sensitivity.

DESSERTS. If you offer your novice eater desserts, chances are he'll readily accept them and even want more. But offering desserts at this stage is not a good idea. Many commercially prepared baby desserts offer little valuable nutrition but lots of sugar. Stick with fruit or yogurt for a sweet taste to top off your baby's meal.

Vitamin and Mineral Supplements

Breastmilk provides complete nutrition for about the first 6 months of life. Infant formulas are developed with the complete vitamin and mineral needs of your infant in mind when exclusive breastfeeding is not possible. After your baby begins the weaning process, however, your pediatrician will check that she's getting enough of the nutrients she needs. The decision whether or not to give a multivitamin or mineral supplement is one you should discuss with your pediatrician. Before you decide, here's what you should know.

Vitamin and mineral products for infants come in the form of liquid drops, which typically contain either vitamins A, D, and C with or without iron, or vitamins A, D, E, and C and the B vitamins thiamin, riboflavin, niacin, and B_6 with or without iron. Both types of vitamin drops can be purchased without a prescription. You won't find the B vitamin folic acid in liquid supplements because it is unstable in liquid form and tends to break down.

The mineral fluoride is another important nutrient. It is critical for the formation of your child's teeth. If you live in an area where the water is not fluoridated, if you give your child only bottled water, or if your drinking water is filtered through a process called reverse osmosis, the American Academy of Pediatrics recommends giving a fluoride-containing supplement between feedings after 6 months of age. Fluoride supplements are available by prescription only, alone or in combination with vitamins. Call your local water company to find out if your water contains fluoride. In some areas, fluoride occurs naturally but the levels may be too low to benefit children's teeth. If your local water is not fluoridated, ask your pediatrician about fluoride supplements.

A healthy infant who is consuming breastmilk or formula along with a variety of solid foods, including good sources of iron and vitamins A and C, shouldn't need supplemental vitamins and minerals. If, however, your infant is at risk for nutrient deficiencies because of chronic health problems that affect his ability to eat, or if his appetite is poor, you should ask your pediatrician whether a supplement is advisable.

? ISSUES PARENTS OFTEN RAISE ABOUT THE TRANSITION TO SOLID FOODS

My pediatrician says to wait to start giving my baby solid foods, but my neighbor's baby is exactly the same age and he's already eating solid foods. Is my baby behind?
Follow your pediatrician's advice. While one child may be ready for solids at 4 months, another may not be ready at 6 months or even older. Both babies are in the "normal range," and your pediatrician will advise you about introducing solids, depending on your baby's rate of development (see p. 23).

At 4 months, my baby still isn't sleeping through the night, and my mother-in-law says that giving him solid foods will fix the problem.
Your mother-in-law means well, but research doesn't back up her opinion. Your baby will be able to sleep for extended periods only when his digestive and nervous systems are mature. Be patient. Your baby will soon be sleeping through the night and switching to solid food. (Read more about the transition on p. 25.)

Why is rice cereal the one that's recommended for starters?
Rice is free of gluten, a protein in some grains that can trigger allergic reactions. A child may also be sensitive to rice cereal, but this is rare. Your pediatrician will advise when it's safe to introduce other grains into your baby's diet. (Also see pp. 24 and 32.)

How many calories does my baby need?
Your baby's calorie needs vary according to how fast he's growing and how active he is. It's important to remember, however, that babies don't eat calories, they eat food, and they regulate their intake according to their needs. (See p. 25.)

Is it really important to introduce foods just one at a time?
More than one taste or texture can be overwhelming to a young baby. Also, if you offer something new at every meal, it can be difficult to identify sensitivity reactions to specific foods, should they occur. One new food every 2 to 3 days is a safe approach for getting started. (See p. 25.)

When my baby switches to cow's milk, can she go straight on to skim?
When your baby switches to cow's milk at about 12 months, she should have whole milk because she needs the fat calories it provides. Starting around your child's second birthday, you can switch to low-fat or fat-free milk. (Also see p. 29).

CHAPTER 3

The Toddler Years

David and Helen Chu thought they had feeding all figured out when baby Andrew smoothly crossed over to solid foods. In fact, by the end of his first year, Andrew was eating any food they offered him and could drink from a cup as if he'd been doing it all his life. He had moved easily from purées to more chunky textures, and now most of his meals were well-chopped servings of what his parents were eating.

Suddenly, however, Andrew had become a toddler and he just wouldn't eat anymore. David and Helen encouraged ("One for Daddy... one for Mommy..."), pleaded ("Just two more bites?"), and threatened ("No cookie if you don't eat up your broccoli!"). No matter what they tried, Andrew always started playing with his food long before the plate was empty. Feeling desperate, they asked their pediatrician, "Where did we go wrong?"

A toddler may gain no more than about 3 to 5 pounds over the whole of his second year, though he probably gained that much in only about 4 months during the first year. From now on, your child will grow at a slower, steadier rate until he reaches the other big growth spurt at puberty. Because he's growing more slowly, he doesn't need to eat as much as he did during his first massive burst of growth.

"Relax," the doctor assured them. "This drop in appetite is a normal stage in development and—at 13 months—Andrew is right on schedule.

"Try giving him smaller portions, with a second helping only if he seems to want more. Don't bargain over foods: If you're serving fruit or yogurt for dessert, just make it part of the meal and let Andrew eat it if he wants to.

"Finally, when he starts playing with his food,

he's letting you know that eating time is over. That's your cue to clear the table and go on to the next activity."

Catch-down Growth

It's normal to feel alarmed when you see a sharp drop in your child's appetite starting around the time of the first birthday. Soon after reaching the one-year milestone, most children are literally toddling everywhere, developing new skills, and getting into all kinds of scrapes as they explore their expanding world. So it's logical to think that an active toddler would need extra food to power this nonstop activity. As if to balance these giant leaps in development, however, the growth rate slows.

Pediatricians refer to this phase as "catch-down growth." It's a process that may start as early as 4 to 6 months and is usually complete by 18 months. Catch-down growth is most clearly seen in a high-birth-weight (9 or 10 pounds) baby whose parents are of average size. While children can be considerably taller and heavier when compared with their parents' size at similar ages, most conform to a general family pattern of growth and size. Thus, after an initial period of fast growth, the child slows down and settles at a level appropriate to the genes he's inherited.

Catch-down growth is the opposite of catch-up growth, which occurs when a child makes up for a setback due to illness.

Who's in Charge?

When you serve food to your children, the responsibility for dealing with it is split two ways. You are in charge of deciding what to offer, and your child is in charge of deciding whether to eat it or not. However, what frequently happens is that the parent announces what's for dinner and the child protests. Then the parent—anxious in case the child doesn't eat enough—backs down

 LOVE ME, LOVE MY FOOD?

When your toddler turns down food, she's not rejecting you. If you stop and reflect for a moment, you'll see that her negativism shows you're doing a good job. Your youngster trusts you enough to say "No," confident that this refusal won't change your love for her. Accept what she tells you.

by asking what the child would like to eat. This line of behavior leads to several outcomes, all of them negative. First, when the parent asks the child what she'd like, it puts the child in the inappropriate role of choosing food for the family. Children don't have the knowledge necessary to make such important choices; it's unfair to expect them to decide what's good for themselves or their families. Second, if more than one child is involved and each has a different request, the parent turns into a short-order cook: "Hamburger for this one...spaghetti for that one...who gets

the omelet?" If a child turns up her nose at what's served, you don't have to apologize or make excuses. All you need to say is, "This is what we're having today." It's a mistake to encourage, persuade, or bribe a child to eat. Research has shown that such efforts have the opposite effect from what's intended, and the child may actually end up eating less than if left alone. If your child refuses the meal you offer, it's not your job to provide an alternative. You probably worry that if your child doesn't eat she'll get hungry. Of course she will! And when she's hungry, she'll eat. There's no better stimulus than hunger for getting a child to try something new. However, if your toddler misses a meal of his own free choice, it won't make him sick and he'll probably be ready to eat at the next regular meal or snacktime. (Or if not the next, then the one after that.)

It's Food, Not Law Enforcement

Keep your priorities in perspective. It's your job, as the adult, to help your toddler learn a healthy eating pattern. This means that you should provide healthful meals at regular times. You also need to prepare the food in forms and textures that she can learn to eat by herself. And you should keep her company during mealtimes so she learns to eat in a safe and socially acceptable way. But you're the food provider, not the food police. At every age, it's up to your child to choose what she wants from the food that's offered, and to decide how much or how little to eat at a meal.

What parents should do is provide appropriate servings of a healthy selection from the Food Guide Pyramid (p. 90), and respect the child's limits. If she says she's had enough, she knows what she's talking about. Don't insist on "just one more mouthful," or make her finish everything.

When it comes to persuading children to eat, pediatricians advise parents to step back: Healthy children don't starve as long as food is available, and attempts to get them to eat more may actually backfire.

It's natural to worry that your child isn't getting enough to eat when she seems to turn down every dish you offer. It's also understandable that you feel let down if your toddler refuses the food you've lovingly prepared.

Whether your toddler just turns her head away from the food or makes a mess with it, keep your comments to a minimum and don't beg or bargain with her. Clean up the mess, offer bread and whatever else is already on the table as an alternative, and, if she turns it down, let her know that mealtime is over. If you ask what she wants or leave the table to whip up something on the spot, you're only setting yourself up for battles that you can't win.

Of course, you should respect your child's likes and dislikes. It's not fair to insist on serving textures and flavors that make her gag. At any given meal, place a reasonable selection on the table, with whole-grain bread or crackers as an option if the main dish doesn't appeal. However, if your child often gags, it may be an indication that she's feeling unbearable pressure to eat. Perhaps it's time to back off and let her take the initiative about eating.

Jason was born with a heart murmur. His pediatrician told Jason's parents that the murmur required no treatment and would disappear as the baby grew. "In a baby with normal growth," the doctor assured them, "a murmur of this type clears up by about 14 months of age."

Jason had few health problems. He began to eat solid foods, in addition to breastmilk, at about 6 months. However, his parents worried because he was smaller than other babies they knew. They were afraid that if he didn't grow enough, the heart murmur would not go away. Each time Jason finished a meal, they urged him to swallow a few more spoonfuls. Jason turned his face away; he knew when he'd had enough and didn't want extra food forced on him. Finally, the parents stopped insisting.

At Jason's one-year checkup, his pediatrician smiled. "Small, yes, but perfectly formed," she said to his parents. "Jason is growing steadily and he's almost walking. His development is fine. Don't worry about his eating. You're right to let him decide how much he wants. This is a boy who knows his own mind!"

Results of studies on children's eating habits show that children are born with the ability to regulate their food intake according to the energy

Foster your toddler's growing independence by letting him make choices, but don't overwhelm him. In other words, limit the possibilities you offer.

Let him take part in preparing the meal and the table. Given a job he can manage, no matter how small it seems to you, your toddler will focus more on his sense of accomplishment and less on the food.

Your toddler is experiencing everything through her senses for the first time. She wants to explore the taste and feel of food not just with her tongue but with her hands as well, just as she loves to squish mud between her toes and let sand run through her fingers. Let her play with the textures and fingerpaint on her tray-table—it only takes a minute to rinse it off in the sink. This phase, like most others, will be over before you know it.

they use. Parents who try to control their child's food intake, or insist on a clean plate at every meal, are interfering with this natural system. A typical example of misguided control is withholding dessert as a punishment for not finishing the vegetables. If you're serving dessert, think of it as neither more nor less important than the broccoli. All parts of the meal should have equal value. Let dessert be just another healthful part of the meal, and don't hold it out as a reward for good behavior.

One way to stop some feeding battles before they start is to let your toddler take part in meal preparation. When you set the table, let him choose between, say, the red cup and the blue. Even if he has a favorite plate or cup of his own, he might like to use a different, "special" one for a change. Put a little milk or juice in a pitcher he can lift and let him pour a drink for himself. Don't worry if most of it ends up on the high-chair tray; your toddler will also enjoy helping to wipe up the mess. A child who dislikes baby bibs may feel more grown up having a cloth napkin tied under his chin.

"I Want to Do It Myself!"

As their muscular coordination steadily improves, toddlers learn to feed themselves. You'll still need to help out for a while and you shouldn't expect neatness at mealtimes for a long time yet. However, the sooner you let your toddler feed herself and get a bit messy, the earlier she'll reach the next stage of development: using utensils properly, quitting the high chair, and joining the rest of the family at the table.

Helping your child eat isn't the same thing as force-feeding with a spoon. Offer help when it's needed, but let your toddler assume increasing responsibility for getting the food from the plate to her mouth. At first, your toddler will eat mainly by finger-feeding. As her coordination improves, she'll enjoy learning to use cutlery. Give her the right tools for the job: unbreakable dishware, a plate with a suction cup that won't slide around the tray-table, a blunt-edge spoon

▶ **EATING TIME IS OVER**

Toddlers have a limited attention span. This applies to eating just as it does to play. If your toddler wants to get down from the table, let her do so. But clear away the plates and don't offer cookies or crackers away from the table to make up for what she didn't eat during the meal. If she's hungry, she'll enjoy her next regularly scheduled snack all the more.

with a handle little fingers can easily grasp, a stubby fork, and a two-handled cup with a firmly fitting, spouted lid.

How Much Does My Toddler Need to Eat?

A toddler's eating habits tend to be unpredictable. One day he may devour enough breakfast for two people, but at later meals, leave his plate almost untouched. The next day, he may eat three square meals plus a couple of snacks.

The amount of food a toddler needs is the amount that keeps up a good rate of growth and energy. Although the average toddler's daily intake rounds off at about 1,000 calories, he doesn't need

 SERVING SIZES FOR TODDLERS

Here's a general guide for feeding your toddler. Each day, a child between ages 1 and 3 needs about 40 calories for every inch of height. This means that a toddler who measures 32 inches, for example, should be taking in an average of about 1,300 calories a day, but the amount varies with each child's build and activity level.

How does this stack up? Your toddler will get enough calories along with all the protein, vitamins, and minerals he needs from an average daily intake similar to the following:

Food group	Servings per day	Number of calories per day	One serving equals
Grains	6 servings	250 calories	Bread, 1/4 to 1/2 slice Cereal, rice, pasta, cooked, 4 tablespoons Cereal, dry, 1/4 cup Crackers, 1 to 2
Vegetables	2 to 3 servings	75 calories	Vegetables, cooked 1 tablespoon for each year of age
Fruits	2 to 3 servings	75 calories	Fruit, cooked or canned, 1/4 cup Fruit, fresh, 1/2 piece Juice, 1/4 to 1/2 cup (2 to 4 ounces)
Dairy	2 to 3 servings	300 to 450 calories	Milk, 1/2 cup Cheese, 1/2 ounce (1-inch cube) Yogurt, 1/3 cup
Protein group: **meat, fish,** **poultry, tofu**	2 servings	200 calories	1 ounce (equal to two 1-inch cubes of solid meat or 2 tablespoons of ground meat) Egg, 1/2 any size, yolk and white
Legumes: **dried beans,** **peas, lentils**	2 servings	200 calories	Soaked and cooked, 2 tablespoons (1/8 cup)
Peanut butter **(smooth only)**		95 calories	1 tablespoon spread thin on bread, toast, or cracker

a fixed number of calories every day, nor do you have to count every calorie he consumes. In fact, children's calorie needs vary widely according to their activity levels and rates of growth and metabolism. If your toddler doesn't eat as much as the child next door—or seems to devour twice as much—it's because his needs are different. Resist the urge to coax another mouthful, and, by the same token, don't forbid a moderate second helping. Studies show that in the long run, coaxing and encouragement have the opposite effect from what is intended. Children are the best judges of how much food they need. You'll develop a sense of how much your toddler is really eating as you serve a regular daily schedule of three small, balanced meals plus a couple of snacks.

What's a Toddler Portion?

A portion for a toddler should be about a quarter of the serving you'd give an adult. Typical serving sizes are 1 to 2 tablespoons of vegetables and about half an ounce—a 1-inch cube—of meat, depending on the child's appetite (see Serving Sizes for Toddlers, p. 41). These servings may seem modest, but it's better to start small and give seconds. Too big a portion can be overwhelming and take away a child's appetite. Starting small allows a greater chance of success, with more opportunities for praise. Keep in mind that when it comes to feeding toddlers, no two days—and no two toddlers—are alike. Appetites and needs vary widely from one child to another and even in the same child from day to day.

Snacks to Stoke the Fire

With all the energy your toddler uses, his stomach can't hold enough to keep him from getting hungry between meals. Many children need a morning and afternoon snack, which should be timed so it won't interfere with lunch or dinner. Snacks should include a satisfying balance of healthful foods.

Raw vegetables are mostly too difficult for toddlers to manage and some—carrots, whole cherry tomatoes, whole green beans, celery—are a serious choking hazard (also see Unsafe for Toddlers, p. 47). But there's no reason that a toddler shouldn't enjoy well-cooked vegetables cut into manageable pieces. Big chunks of any food and globlike spoonfuls of peanut butter are hazardous and should not be given to children younger than age 4. They don't yet have the ability to chew with the grinding motion that reduces food to a consistency safe for swallowing.

The Toddler's Diet: A Balancing Act

You don't have to include the exact number of daily servings from each Food Guide Pyramid group at every meal or snack. The idea is to provide a varied diet that includes a good amount from each group when averaged out over a 2-week period. If you follow the general guide in Serving Sizes for Toddlers, (p. 41), your toddler will get a good balance of grains and cereals; vegetables and fruits; meat, fish, eggs; and dairy products.

Keep the Menu Simple

Young children prefer simple foods. Don't wear yourself out making elaborate recipes to tempt a picky toddler. Your child is experiencing many foods for the first time. Heavy seasonings and sauces only obscure the taste and may put a toddler off the food.

Young children also tend to be more comfortable with what they know, including food. It's easy to sympathize with this conservative tendency when you consider how many things a toddler has to face for the first time and the many

Fresh fruits		Apples, bananas, peaches, nectarines, pears (sliced) Cherries, grapes, plums (sliced and pitted) Orange or grapefruit sections (cut into pieces) Strawberries
Dried fruits		Apples, apricots, peaches, pears (cut up) Dates, prunes (pitted, cut up) Raisins
Vegetables		Carrots, green beans (well cooked, diced) Steamed cauliflower, broccoli Yams (cooked and diced) Peas (mashed for safety; a child can inhale whole peas) Potatoes (cooked and diced)
Dairy products		Cheese (grated or diced) Cottage cheese Yogurt, fresh or frozen Milk
Breads and cereals		Whole-wheat bread Bagel cut into small pieces Crackers (saltine, graham, whole grain) Dry cereal Pretzels Rice cakes
Meat/protein group		Fish (canned tuna, salmon, sardines; whitefish) Peanut butter (smooth, spread thin on bread or cracker)

new activities he masters in remarkably few attempts. This is one reason why fast-food chains, with their standardized menus, are magnets for families. Customers know exactly what they're getting—"When you've eaten at one restaurant in a chain, you've eaten at them all."

There's nothing wrong with serving the same food day in, day out, if that's what your toddler prefers. It's a lot easier to achieve balanced nutrition, however, if you vary the menu. Parents may think of their child as a creature of habit because he has a peanut butter and jelly sandwich for lunch come rain or come shine. Often, it's the parents who have established the habit. Try to introduce reasonable variety with a rotating schedule of dinner dishes, different snacks, and new breakfast foods from time to time.

New Foods: A Little at a Time

When you introduce a new food, you may find that it's best to place no more than a teaspoonful on the plate alongside a favorite food until your toddler gets used to it. At every age, it's best to serve a small portion and give a second helping if the child asks for more. The sight of a plate heaped with food can overwhelm a young child.

The parents of a toddler learn to take nothing for granted, especially when it comes to eating. Toddlers are notorious for food fads and food strikes. Don't make an issue of them; instead, simply let your child choose from what's on the table. If he repeatedly refuses a particular food, give it a rest, then reintroduce it, without comment, after a few weeks. Or serve it again when your toddler asks for it and it fits into your meal plan.

If he insists on the same food several days in a row, there's no harm in serving it provided it's nourishing and healthful. Place a small helping of something new or different alongside the favorite; sooner or later he'll try it.

Though it's up to parents and caregivers to schedule meals and vary the menu to ensure a good balance, it's the child's job to decide how much to eat and, indeed, whether he's going to eat at all. At times, young children are unwilling to eat because they don't feel hungry.

Four-year-old Nicole wasn't interested in eating when the family sat down to a hot dog lunch. Her mother wrapped Nicole's hot dog in foil and put it in the refrigerator. At snack time 2 hours later, Nicole retrieved her now-cold hot dog. She declined her mother's offer to warm it up and, instead, ate it "as is" with real enjoyment.

Far better to skip a meal than to risk a standoff with bad feelings on both sides of the table. Whether you're a child or a grownup, food is always more appealing when you're really hungry.

Fear of Trying

As if eating less, pickiness, and food jags weren't enough to deal with, many parents find themselves across the table from a person with conservative views about food. You make something new and serve it up to your 2-year-old, certain that the color and aroma will pique her appetite. But with arms crossed and teeth clenched, she stares straight ahead like a face on Mount Rushmore. Nothing will induce her to eat.

When it comes to food, children at the toddler stage know what they're comfortable with. They mistrust the very idea of trying something new, no matter how much trouble you took to make it and how good you think it looks and tastes.

Without drawing unnecessary attention to it, let your child see you eating and enjoying the new food. Your child will learn from your example.

▷ **FOOD FADS AND JAGS**

A 2-year-old on a food jag may insist on the same food 10, 20, or 30 days in a row. On the 11th, 21st, or 31st day, however, he'll make a face at the food he used to cry for and say, "I don't eat that!" According to toddler reasoning, he's right. In his mind, he used to eat it (maybe…), but he doesn't anymore.

> You can't force a new food on a toddler. Instead, try a soft-sell approach by serving a very small portion alongside an established favorite when the child is hungry.

Food Strikes and Mealtime Wars

Refusing food brings a fast, emotional response from parents that the toddler interprets as caring attention. Toddlers enjoy extra time and focus from their parents.

Toddlers often choose mealtimes to put on a show of independence. This is extremely trying for a parent who has put time and effort—not to mention imagination—into preparing a meal. To make it worse, these wildcat actions often take place at the end of a tiring work day or when you're caught up with the needs of others in the family. Quick to pick up new habits, toddlers soon learn that refusing food is an effective way to get attention.

Treat food refusals matter-of-factly and keep the conversation on subjects other than food. Above all, don't resort to spoon-feeding and begging your child to eat. Researchers studying children's eating patterns found that when parents coaxed, pleaded, and insisted, children ate less than when they were left to eat at their own pace.

No Liquid Lunches

Some toddlers drink so much milk and juice that they have no appetite when it's time for more nourishing meals and snacks. Also, children who drink a lot of juice can develop toddler diarrhea (the fruit sugar fructose and sorbitol, a sugar that is not absorbed, can cause diarrhea). With this condition, an otherwise healthy child passes numerous semiliquid bowel movements, usually containing fairly large amounts of undigested food, over the course of the day. Toddler diarrhea is not a serious health problem. All important nutrients are absorbed, and weight gain continues normally.

Milk is an important and inexpensive source of necessary fats, protein, calcium, and vitamins A and D. However, a toddler doesn't need more than 16 to 24 ounces (two to three average glasses) of milk a day. Your child's appetite for meals may improve if you offer water instead of juice when she's thirsty. Water is more thirst-quenching than sugary drinks such as juice. Juices do supply some vitamin C, which either occurs naturally in citrus juices or may be added, as in apple juice. Also, calcium-fortified orange juice is a good source of calcium. However, giving juices can be a rather expensive way to provide these nutrients. Juices mainly provide calories that the toddler can get in a more nourishing form from solid foods.

If you tell your toddler there's no juice available and offer water instead, he'll drink it without

> One study showed that children did not accept a new food until they'd been served it an average of 10 times. (By that time, it was an old food.) Some accepted it earlier, but many had to see it even more than 10 times. So, if at first you don't succeed, don't give up: Keep offering small servings. Sooner or later, your young child will work the food into her routine.

protest. Alternatively, you may cut down gradually over a week or two by giving a slightly smaller serving each time he asks for juice and diluting it with increasing amounts of water.

Don't be concerned that you're depriving your child of calcium and vitamins if you cut her milk consumption to a limit of 16 to 24 ounces per day. She'll get plenty from other dairy products and foods in a balanced diet (check the sources of vitamins and minerals in the chart on p. 97).

Lights! Food! Action!

Some parents are so anxious about feeding that they feel driven to provide diversions such as toys and videos during meals. Food is nourishment, not entertainment, and you don't have to turn your dining area into a theme restaurant to get your child to eat. In the long run, such measures can prove counterproductive. Your child may find it difficult to eat without distractions and may not learn socially acceptable behavior.

Turn the television off when it's time to eat, and clear away toys, reading materials, and other distractions. Encourage your children to express their opinions and take part in the conversation at mealtimes.

Make family mealtimes special, although you don't have to turn every dinner into a major production. Sit down to eat with your toddler. Serve meals at the table, not in front of the television. Even your toddler's snacks should be served at a special place, not eaten on the run. Avoid serving snacks while children are watching television.

▷ **PHASING OUT BOTTLES**

A toddler who is still drinking from a bottle may skip meals if he knows the bottle is available. Encourage your child to drink from a cup. When you serve juice, for example, always serve it in a cup. Bottles should be phased out between 12 and 24 months.

This habit can lead to unconscious overeating and unwanted weight gain later in life.

Food Safety

Choking on food is a serious hazard that's all too common among toddlers. Lumps of food can easily lodge in a little throat and block the airway. Children don't learn to chew with a grinding motion until about age 4. That's why firm, smooth foods such as nuts and hard candies are so dangerous for children younger than 4. They simply don't have the ability to chew them well. Choking often happens when a toddler tries to do everything at once, eating as he runs or talks. If a toddler likes the taste of something, he may try to stuff the entire portion into his mouth until his cheeks bulge like a chipmunk's and he can't move his jaw to chew and swallow properly. Especially risky are hard foods, such as raw carrots and celery; foods with a resistant, rubbery texture, such as large chunks of boiled waxy potatoes; round, firm foods; hot dogs and other meat; and thick lumps of firm, "gloppy" spreads, such as peanut butter. Foods can generally be considered safe if they dissolve in the saliva: for example, graham crackers, cereal, and pasta. Take other preventive steps as follows:

- Chop food to a texture that's easy for a young child to manage.
- Don't let your toddler eat while running or playing.
- Make sure that older children don't give unsuitable foods to a toddler.

- Never leave your toddler alone while eating.
- Teach your toddler to finish a mouthful before speaking.
- Keep an eye on your toddler whether you're eating with him or not: A choking child may be unable to make any sound at all.

Pouching

David, at 18 months, ate a relatively limited range of foods and disliked meat, but was growing well and had plenty of energy. His parents weren't concerned, as they were confident he'd eventually enjoy a wider variety, just as his elder brother did.

When David was served a hamburger at a barbecue lunch hosted by family friends, the toddler took a large bite and chewed it for a long time. Unwilling to swallow the detested meat, but anxious to be a well-mannered guest, David pouched the hamburger in his cheeks and resisted all suggestions that he swallow or spit it out. At bedtime that evening, his mother, worried that the toddler could choke, begged and pleaded to no avail. Finally, she gently pinched David's nostrils and he immediately sprayed her with a stream of chewed-up hamburger, to his brother's delight.

Although David's mother hadn't actually forced food on him, she recalled that she had warned him several times to "be a good boy at the barbecue." David interpreted this as an order to eat. Despite his mother's good intentions, David felt pressure and resisted in the most tactful way he could, by pouching. He would allow the food he didn't like into his mouth but no farther.

It's not unusual for toddlers to leave the table with food in their mouths. Some children chew for a while, then spit out the food. Others wad it up in their cheeks for hours until they look like chipmunks. A child who pouches in this way may take more than he wants just to satisfy a parent who insists on "one more mouthful." Some children also dislike the taste or texture of certain foods or are afraid to swallow.

▶ UNSAFE FOR TODDLERS

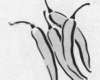

- Hot dogs (unless cut in quarters lengthwise before being sliced)
- Hard candies, including jelly beans
- Nuts
- Chunks of peanut butter—peanut butter may be spread thinly on bread or cracker—never give chunks of peanut butter to a toddler
- Popcorn
- Raw carrots, celery, green beans
- Seeds (such as processed pumpkin or sunflower seeds)
- Whole grapes, cherry tomatoes (cut them in quarters)
- Large chunks of any food such as meat, potatoes, or raw vegetables and fruits

If your child is **CHOKING** and can't breathe, have somebody call the Emergency Medical Service (**911**) while you start the following emergency measures. But if the child is coughing, crying, or speaking, **DO NOT** do any of the following; instead call the EMS (911) or your pediatrician for advice.

For a Choking 1- to 3-year-old:

1. Lay the child on his back.

2. Kneel at the child's feet or stand if he's on a raised surface, place the heel of one hand on the middle of the child's abdomen above the navel and below the ribcage. Place your other hand over the first.

3. Press into the abdomen with up to 5 rapid upward thrusts. Keep thrusts gentle in a small child.

4. Lift jaw and tongue forward with your thumb and index finger. If you can see the food, sweep it out with your other index finger.

Repeat steps 2 and 3 until the child coughs up the food, starts to breathe, or becomes unconscious.

   If the child becomes unconscious, give mouth-to-mouth resuscitation until emergency help arrives.

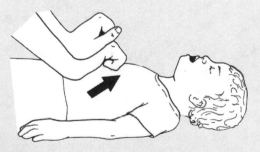

Heimlich Maneuver for an Older Child

1. Treat a choking older child standing, sitting, or lying down.

2. From behind the child, place the thumbside of a fist against the middle of the child's abdomen, just above the navel. Grasp the fist with your other hand.

3. Give up to 5 firm, rapid, upward thrusts into the abdomen.

Repeat steps 2 and 3 until the child coughs up the food, starts to breathe, or becomes unconscious.

   If the child becomes unconscious, give mouth-to-mouth resuscitation until emergency help arrives.

Risks associated with pouching include choking (if a wad becomes dislodged) and tooth decay (if the child is in the habit of pouching carbohydrates for long periods). If your child will cooperate, the best way to deal with pouching is simply to ask him to spit out or swallow the food, or to clear out the food yourself with your finger. If all else fails, a last resort is to lightly pinch the nostrils. Most important in the long run, think about how you communicate with your child, to make sure you're not putting pressure on him to eat.

Where Does Fat Fit In?

Young children need calories from fat for growth and brain development. This is especially important in the first 2 years of life. Even as adults, we all need a moderate amount of fat to supply energy, to keep our skin healthy and supple, to help wounds heal, and to keep our hair growing thick and shiny. Fat helps us absorb certain vitamins that are essential for health. It also adds flavor and a pleasing texture to foods.

However, too much fat can add to our risk of developing heart disease, the leading cause of death in the United States and other developed countries. We can reduce the risk of heart disease by cutting down on excessive fat in the diet from childhood onward.

Although babies should get half of all their calories from fat, nutrition experts recommend that after age 2, children's diets should be gradually modified until they are getting about one third of their daily calories from fat. This is the same fraction advised for adults, so it's a fairly simple matter to keep the whole family on a low-fat program. It's especially important to do so if heart disease runs in the family.

After age 2, you can switch your toddler to skim or low-fat milk, like the rest of the family.

Help your children to develop a preference for low-fat foods. As they approach kindergarten age, start buying fat-free yogurt. Serve cheese in moderate portions and select cheeses made from skim milk. Goat's milk cheeses and yogurts are lower in

▷ **TO REDUCE FAT CALORIES**

INSTEAD OF...	SERVE...
Hamburgers, hot dogs	Lean chicken, fish, vegetable "burgers"
French fries, processed potato nuggets, instant potatoes made with butter or margarine	Baked potatoes, home-made oven fries, mashed or scalloped potatoes made with low-fat yogurt or buttermilk
Fried chicken and fish, commercial breaded chicken and fish preparations	Baked or grilled chicken and fish
Doughnuts, Danish pastries, croissants, toaster cakes	Whole-grain bread, bagels, English muffins
Chocolate-chip cookies, frosted cupcakes, brownies	Graham crackers, fat-free fig bars, oatmeal-date cookies
Ice cream, milkshakes	Sherbet, ice milk, nonfat frozen yogurt, juice popsicles, fruit and yogurt shakes

saturated fats than most cow's milk products (read more about the different types of fats in Chapter 6); compare labels. For frozen treats, sherbets, juice popsicles without added sugar, and nonfat frozen yogurt are more healthful than ice cream.

You can cut down on dietary fat by substituting lower-fat for higher-fat foods (such as grilled fish for a hamburger) or serving a reduced-fat version of a food (broiled fish instead of deep-fried, breaded fillets).

Treats or Tricks

A treat of potato chips, ice cream, or candy now and then won't do any harm, but there's no need to put temptation in your child's way. Don't keep large containers of ice cream in your freezer or giant bags of cookies and salty snacks in the pantry. Buy or make small batches only for treats on special occasions. Then, when your child asks, you can honestly reply, "There aren't any in the house," and offer fresh fruit, a vegetable snack, or whole-grain crackers instead.

Nutritional Supplements: Save Your Money

Vitamin and mineral deficiencies are rare in the United States, even among those who are eating poorly balanced diets. That's because many of our basic foods—breads, cereals, rice, milk, and margarine—are fortified with vitamins, minerals, or both.

Like many consumers, you may do a quick calculation as you scan food labels to make sure that what your child is eating will cover the Recommended Dietary Allowances (RDAs) of vitamins and minerals. Health authorities are now recommending that we get an Adequate Daily Intake of nutrients. The name may have changed, but the levels are close to the old RDAs and the purpose is the same: to safeguard health.

The RDAs are set well above the amounts we actually need. A balanced diet based on the Food Guide Pyramid supplies more than enough vitamins and minerals for every age group. A toddler who is getting the right number of daily servings from the various food groups—even in very small portions—will always get enough of these essential nutrients.

Our bodies use vitamins to convert food into energy, and minerals, such as calcium, are necessary for building bone and muscle. The small amounts we need are obtained from a normal diet.

Advertisements and promotions for processed food and supplements try to plant the idea that our children's diets lack vitamins and minerals. They put pressure on families to use supplements as a kind of insurance against nutritional shortfalls. These claims are written not by health professionals but by ad writers who work to sell the products. Most children do not need vitamin or mineral supplements. Healthy people retain only as much of the water-soluble vitamins (vitamin C and the B vitamins) as they need; the rest passes out in the urine. The other supplement story—which the ads don't bother to tell—is that too much of a good thing can be bad. For example, vitamins A and D are fat soluble and are stored in the tissues. When excessively high doses are taken, the tissue stores can build up to toxic levels and make people sick. High doses of iron, zinc, and other minerals taken over a prolonged period can accumulate in the body and may have adverse effects on the digestive tract, liver, heart, kidneys and other organs.

On the whole, healthy people absorb only as much of most water-soluble vitamins as they need; any extra is excreted in the urine. So spending money on supplements is not only costly but also wasteful.

Pills and potions won't make up for a poor diet. If a young child is undernourished or has problems related to an inadequate diet, what's needed is a change in eating habits or the kind of food that's provided, not neccessarily supplements. In conditions such as chronic illness where a child can't eat enough, is unable to absorb certain nutrients, or has a sensitivity to certain foods, pediatricians may prescribe supplements to meet special needs. In general, however, give your child supplements only if your pediatrician advises you to do so.

FOOD PROBLEMS THAT TODDLERS' PARENTS OFTEN WORRY ABOUT

No matter what I put on the table, my toddler says, "No!"
This resistance is just a normal sign of growing independence. Continue providing regular, healthful meals and snacks and let your toddler choose what to eat and how much at a time. (See p. 38.)

How much does my toddler need to eat?
Most young children do well with three small meals and two snacks daily. The guideline is about 40 calories a day for every inch of height, or about 1,000 calories a day for the average toddler, but appetites vary among children and in the same child from day to day. (See p. 41 for recommended servings.)

Does each meal have to include every food group?
Base your toddler's meals on the Food Guide Pyramid, so that the overall intake balances out over the course of 2 weeks or so. (See Chapter 6.)

How much milk does my toddler need?
Two or three 6- to 8-ounce glasses a day is about right. Offer water when your child is thirsty and don't overdo milk and juice between meals. (Check p. 45 for more about toddlers and liquids.)

When is the right time to cut down on fat?
Children should get about half their daily calories from fat up to age 2. After that, cut down gradually, until the diet supplies about one-third of daily calories from fat between ages 4 and 5. This is also the percentage recommended for adults. (See p. 49.)

My toddler never finishes a plateful of food.
Serve smaller portions. Your child is growing more slowly than in the first year of life and doesn't need to eat so much. You can always give a second helping if your toddler asks for it. (See p. 37.)

CHAPTER 4

Nutrition During the School Years

When Lauren Maier found herself juggling pots and pans to cook an alternative main course for the umpteenth time, a light finally went on: "This is my house, my family. I cook the dinner and I call the shots. Let's make ourselves happy."

She stopped asking the children what they wanted to eat. Instead, she prepared food and served it without comment. To Lauren's surprise, her 4- and 6-year-olds quickly adjusted to the new system. When they objected to the food they found on their plates, they could always fill up on the whole-grain bread and raw vegetable sticks she usually served as part of the meal. Lauren stopped wheedling, pleading, and begging if the children didn't seem to eat much. She remembered what her pediatrician had said: "It may not seem like much to you, but it's enough for a 4-year-old or 6-year-old. You wouldn't want to be force-fed, would you?" As tension around eating decreased, Lauren began to look forward to meals as a relaxing, stimulating time of the day, instead of a test of wills that ended in tears and time-outs.

Choosing Food: A Job for Grownups

The family kitchen is no place for short-order cooking or bargaining over food. As in a restaurant kitchen, one person has to be the chef and make the decisions. In overwhelming numbers,

During the middle years there's an average increase in height of a little more than 2 inches a year for both boys and girls. The corresponding weight gain is about 6 1/2 pounds a year. These numbers, however, are only averages. Heredity, nutrition, and general health are only a few of the many factors that influence your child's growth rate.

parents buy the food and decide what's available in their home. Thus, although children may choose what to eat at various times, they can only select from the food that's offered. Parents decide what to buy, and parents, therefore, determine what children eat.

Mealtimes are social occasions that provide important opportunities for families to talk and share the events of the day. Even if your child doesn't like the food that's served, you should still expect her to join the rest of the family at the table. Let her help herself to bread, salad, and whatever else is on the table, but don't offer an alternative food in place of the dish she has turned down. If she's hungry later, offer to reheat the leftovers or suggest another healthy choice. The one food you shouldn't offer is the alternative she originally demanded.

Children as Educated Consumers

During the school years children are bombarded with TV advertising. About half the ads that children see on TV are for processed foods, and most of the foods are high in fat and simple sugars but low in fiber and protein. Explain to your children that an ad is designed to get them to buy the product, even though it may not be a healthy choice. Help them learn not to be gullible consumers, swayed by promotional pitches. Explain how a food budget works. Finally, keep in mind that there's one fail-safe defense against TV: You can turn it off and organize alternative activities.

Supermarket shelves are stacked on purpose with heavily advertised, high-profit items at children's eye level. That's why it's a good idea to write out a shopping list at home and keep to it. If you find yourself giving in to demands for "this" cereal or "those" cookies just for the sake of peace and quiet, have someone else mind your children so you can shop without being distracted. For example, you could trade shopping time and childcare with a neighbor to help both of you cope. Older children may enjoy helping out in the supermarket. Equip them with a list of items and challenge them to compare brands for nutrient content and unit price, then pick the best values.

Too Many Children Are Not Eating Well

While Americans may enjoy the most abundant and economical food supply in the world, a survey by government health experts revealed worrisome patterns of eating in children and adolescents ranging in age from 2 to 19 years. Fewer than one third of the young people surveyed were consuming the daily servings of grains, fruits, lean meats, and dairy products recommended in the Food Guide Pyramid (see p. 90), while only just over a third were getting the recommended daily servings of vegetables. At least one child in six was not getting the right number of servings in any food group at all. Those who weren't getting the recommended number of servings also failed, not surprisingly, to obtain the Recommended Dietary Allowances (RDAs) for many essential vitamins and minerals. Even for the one child out of one hundred who was getting the right number of servings in all food groups, fat intake was above the recommended limit, because meats weren't

trimmed of fat and whole-milk dairy products were used. No matter which group they were in, all the young people surveyed were eating too much fat and too much added sugar.

Base your children's meals on the Food Guide Pyramid to make sure of a healthful, balanced diet. To keep fat consumption low:

- Trim all fat from meat before cooking.
- Use cooking methods that require little or no fat, such as broiling, steaming, and roasting.
- Switch to skim or low-fat milk and dairy foods for children older than 2.

Promote your family's intake of fiber and vitamins by providing plenty of vegetables and fruits. If your children balk at unadorned vegetables and fruits, try incorporating more of these foods into favorite recipes. For example, you can mix applesauce in waffle batter or mix blueberries or sliced bananas into pancakes. Replace the ground meat in spaghetti sauce or taco filling with a mixture of minced and chopped vegetables, such as onion, carrot, celery, mushrooms, zucchini, squash, and eggplant. For a change from the usual snacks, let your children make their own colorful kebabs with raw fruit chunks and diced cheese, or serve raw vegetable sticks with low-fat dips.

When in Rome . . .

While you're doing your best to keep the healthy-food flag flying, there'll be times during play-dates and sleep-overs when your child has foods you'd never serve at home. What's more, he'll probably enjoy them and tell you so. Relax: An occasional lapse isn't going to wreck the healthy foundation you've laid. Besides, the emotional benefit your child gains from spending time with a friend counts for much more than any potential harm done by a few fatty or nutrient-poor meals.

Compliment your child for having the good manners to eat what he was offered even though it wasn't the kind of food he's used to—and continue to serve healthful meals at home.

Bigger, Not Better

As you stroll through any suburban mall or amusement park, you may notice that many young people look as if their diets are based on quantity rather than quality. For reasons that aren't altogether clear, children are getting heavier, perhaps because they're eating too much and exercising too little.

To meet a surge in the demand for fashionable clothing for overweight children, several major retail chains have added new extra-large sizes to their children's-wear lines and are making some of their regular sizes fuller than they used to. Besides pressing retailers for larger clothes, however, parents who recognize that their children are overweight should also develop ways to help them control their weight. Paying attention to food choices and becoming more active is a proven way to control weight. One approach to help your family stay slim and cut the risk of many illnesses in later life is by following the recommendations of the Food Guide Pyramid (p. 90).

Main dishes should emphasize complex carbohydrates such as brown rice, beans, and pasta. Properly prepared and served in moderate portions, these foods are good, low-fat sources of protein and other nutrients. The body has to work hard to digest them, and they are less likely to promote weight gain than high-fat foods. Switch to skim milk and other low-fat dairy products. For treats, serve sherbets, frozen juice popsicles without added sugar, and nonfat frozen yogurts instead of ice cream. Join your child in regular, moderate exercise such as walking, bicycling, or swimming. Discourage snacking while watching television, which can lead to a habit of overeating.

The key factor in weight regulation is the bal-

▷ **WHAT YOU SEE IS WHAT YOU EAT**

While it's true that children have an inborn ability to regulate their calorie intake according to their needs for growth and energy, they may not always get the calories from the most healthful and nutritious foods. Researchers who studied children's food choices many years ago claimed that children instinctively balanced their diets. But the children were allowed to choose only from an array of fresh, unprocessed foods without added seasonings, sugars, flavor enhancers, or artificial dyes. These young children were not given cookies, candy, potato chips, or other nutrient-poor foods.

In today's world, children are exposed to many commercial foods that try to cover up their poor nutritional quality with advertisements claiming they're "fun to eat." That's why you should get into the habit of comparing the nutritional value of foods served at home and at school with the recommendations of the Food Guide Pyramid. Food labels are an essential source of information. To keep healthy nutrition in focus, educate your children to choose healthful foods for themselves when you aren't around.

ance between the total daily calorie consumption and the amount of energy expended. However, the composition of the diet may also play a role. A study of 9- and 10-year-olds disclosed that boys and girls who ate a lot of fat had more body fat than those whose diet was high in carbohydrates. Even when the young people were eating the same number of calories and getting the same amount of exercise, those in the high-fat-consumption group were carrying more body fat than those who ate more carbohydrates. In this group of children, fatness was related only to diet; it didn't matter whether they were girls or boys, how physically fit they were, or how fat their parents were. (For more information about overweight in children, including how to tell if your child is overweight, see Chapter 8.)

Karen remained an unwavering size 6 by means of constant dieting. She was also determined to protect her daughter Alison from the taunts that had made Karen miserable throughout a chubby childhood and adolescence. Karen never cooked from scratch. With just two in the family, she found it simpler to let Alison choose from frozen dinners at the supermarket and managed her own weight with frozen, calorie-controlled diet entrées. She and Alison also ate out several times a week. After a long day at work, Karen often complained, "I'm too tired to zap anything!" and chose greens from the salad bar while Alison ordered pizza or a double cheeseburger.

Alarmed at Alison's noticeable weight gain as puberty approached, Karen redoubled her efforts and replaced the sweet snacks Alison preferred with fat-free cookies, low-fat ice cream and frozen yogurt, fat-free toppings, and other reduced-fat substitutes. At Alison's next checkup, Karen expressed her concerns: "I keep her on fat-free everything and still she doesn't lose weight."

Their pediatrician explained that fat-free does not mean low in calories; many reduced-fat foods, for example, are high in both sugar and calories. Alison's minor weight gain was not unusual in an adolescent. The best way for both mother and daughter to keep trim was to eat a balanced diet, with plenty of fresh vegetables and fruits. He suggested that Karen try making more meals from basic ingredients and involve Alison

▷ **DO OVERWEIGHT CHILDREN GROW UP OVERWEIGHT?**

For the most part, chubby children under age 3 whose parents are not overweight are likely to trim down as they grow, without further action. However, at any stage of childhood, having an obese parent increases the risk of being overweight as an adult. Cutting calories is not the right approach for children, who need a balance of nutrients for growth. Dietary modifications for young children should never be used except under your pediatrician's close guidance. Your pediatrician can suggest measures to prevent overweight that are aimed at altering the family lifestyle. Such measures will emphasize a sensible diet and regular physical activity.

Any child who has a drastic weight change, whether upward or downward, should be seen by a pediatrician.

in the preparation. He pointed out that a dinner of fresh pasta with vegetable sauce from the refrigerated section was hardly more trouble than juggling different frozen entrées. Premixed greens from the produce display could make a quick salad. Finally, he suggested that both Karen and Alison restrict their TV viewing time and, instead, keep up a program of regular, moderate exercise to use up calories.

If your child is overweight, don't try to put him or her on a weight-loss diet. Instead, see your pediatrician for advice.

Starches to Center Stage

After infancy, children should get about half of their daily calories from carbohydrates, especially starchy foods like whole-grain breads and cereals, beans and rice, potatoes, and pasta. Less emphasis should be placed on sugars, which are simple carbohydrates.

If less than 50 percent of children's calories come from carbohydrates, their plates may be overloaded with meat, cheese, and other foods high in protein and fat. Too much fat in childhood adds to the risk of heart disease and other disorders later on.

Protein: How Much Do Children Need?

Protein is needed for growth as well as to maintain muscle, bone and cartilage, teeth, and every system in the body (also see Chapter 6). As a primary constituent of muscle and bone, protein provides structural support. However, protein is so abundant in the foods Americans eat that most of us, children and adults alike, consume more than we need. Protein overload may be a more serious problem than protein deficiency. While it's important to eat enough protein, researchers believe that eating *too much* protein over many

▶ **PROTEIN RDAs WITH SOURCES AND SERVINGS BASED ON AGE AND WEIGHT**

Age	Child's weight (pounds)	RDA protein (grams/day)	Protein sources	Protein content (grams)
1–3	29	16	Whole milk (1 cup)	8
			Bread, whole wheat (1 slice)	3
4–6	44	22	Egg, boiled (1 large)	6.25
			Cheese, cheddar (1 ounce)	7
7–10	61	28	Macaroni and cheese (1 cup)	17
			Corn muffin (1 medium)	21
			Bagel (1 medium)	7
11–14 (boys)	99	45	Tuna salad (1/2 cup)	16
			Peanut butter (1 tablespoon)	5
			Baked beans (1/2 cup)	9
11–14 (girls)	101	46	Chicken breast, roasted, skinless (half)	27
			English muffin (1 medium)	5

years may contribute to kidney disease and osteoporosis. What's more, our main sources of high-quality (complete) protein are animal products, such as meat and dairy foods, which have a relatively high saturated-fat content. Thus, a diet that includes more protein than necessary may also be too high in fat.

Children require more protein, given their size, than adults because young people need it for growth as well as tissue repair. (See table, p. 57, for a guide to protein requirements.)

Vitamins and Minerals

Surveys indicate that about a quarter of all school-age American children are given vitamin and mineral supplements. These products are seldom necessary. A healthy child eating a balanced diet based on the Food Guide Pyramid should meet the RDAs for all essential vitamins and minerals. (See Chapter 6 for where we get vitamins and what they do.) There's no evidence that levels higher than the RDA are beneficial for healthy children; on the contrary, excessive doses of minerals and high doses, or megadoses, of vitamins A, D, and C can be harmful.

If a child's diet isn't healthy to start with, vitamin and mineral supplements won't make it right. These supplements can't help a child who is regularly consuming too many calories, too much fat, too much sugar, and not enough fiber.

In unusual cases, pediatricians may prescribe supplements. For example, children in homes where a strict vegetarian diet is followed, or children with medical conditions such as cystic fibrosis or malabsorption due to liver or gastrointestinal disease, may require supplements. However, these products should not be used except on your pediatrician's advice.

If you have a picky eater in your family, you may have to juggle the food groups slightly in order to ensure adequate vitamin and mineral intakes, but this is a simple matter of adjusting portions. It's not necessary to spend money on expensive commercial products. (Read more

▷ **EXCHANGING VITAMIN AND MINERAL SOURCES**

Vitamins For children who don't like vegetables	Vitamin A: apricots, cantaloupe, mango, peaches, plums, prunes; milk; eggs. Vitamin C: grapefruit, oranges, cantaloupe and other melons, strawberries.
Calcium For children who don't drink milk	Part-skim and low-fat cheeses, yogurt; broccoli, dark-green leafy vegetables; chickpeas, lentils; canned sardines, salmon, and other fish with bones; calcium-fortified orange juice. Some pediatricians recommend an over-the-counter antacid containing calcium carbonate.
Protein For children who don't eat meat	Lentils, tofu; beans, and other legumes in combination with grains; peanut butter; eggs; fish; nuts; dairy foods.

Studies in large numbers of school-age children have shown that the nutrients most often lacking in their diets are calcium, iron, zinc, vitamin A, vitamin C (ascorbic acid), folic acid, and vitamin B_6 (also called pyridoxine). However, these essential nutrients are so plentiful in foods that a child only needs to consume the minimum number of servings recommended in the Food Guide Pyramid (see p. 90) to get the right amount each day. The missing nutrients can be obtained from the following sources and servings:

Whole grains, fortified cereals, and breads	6 servings	Iron, zinc, vitamin B_6, folic acid
Fruits	2 servings	Vitamins A, B_6, C, folic acid
Milk, cheese, yogurt group	3 servings	Calcium, zinc, vitamins A, B_6
Meat, fish, poultry group	2 servings	Iron, zinc, vitamin B_6
Vegetables (dark yellow; leafy greens; potatoes)	2 servings	Vitamins A, B_6, C, folic acid

about dealing with feeding difficulties and picky eaters on p. 65.)

How Children Act and Eat at School Age

A child of early school age can be a pretty reasonable person; toddler tantrums are forgotten and adolescent turbulence is still a long way off. Most children at this age are prepared to sample a variety of foods. Their appetites vary according to their growth and activity levels. The pattern children establish as toddlers—three full meals and a couple of snacks daily—should continue as they move into the school years.

Maintaining the trend that began around the first birthday, growth keeps up steadily, without the dramatic surges seen in infants and adolescents. Nevertheless, surges do occur. Many parents claim that their school-age children go through phases of "stretching" and "consolidating"—looking alternately lanky and squat. Their appetites may vary in the same way: They may devour everything in sight for a month or so, then cut back as if to make up for it.

As puberty approaches, growth picks up and weight gain may increase to 9 or 10 pounds a year. The normal ranges for girls and boys from 2 to 18 years are shown in the standard growth charts in Appendix III. As the ranges indicate, it's not unusual for preadolescent young people of the same age to differ up to 5 inches in height.

Does Breakfast Really Matter?

Breakfast is the meal that's most likely to get lost in the daily shuffle. Time is short in the morning, even in the best-run households, and many children—especially the "owls" who tend to fall asleep later and make up for it by being harder to rouse in the morning—don't feel like eating during the short time available between getting up and leaving for school. Nevertheless, breakfast is important for a good start. Studies have shown that children who don't eat breakfast have trouble staying alert and concentrating during the first hours of the school day.

If breakfast is your family's stumbling block, you may have to work on both scheduling and meal delivery. Move as many of the morning chores as you can to the evening before and push bedtime up

As their sense of independence grows, school-age children gain a sense of self-worth from doing worthwhile jobs. The problem is, it's sometimes difficult to find jobs that aren't too hazardous or complicated for the age level.

The kitchen is a great place for children to perform tasks that show real results. Cooking is important: Both girls and boys should be taught how to plan and prepare healthful meals. Best of all, cooking jobs start with simple skills that a preschooler can manage, and go right up the scale to high professional levels. Toddlers love to tear salad leaves, stir mixtures, and roll dough. Many little ones learn numbers as their parents count off the eggs, spoonfuls, and cupfuls in recipes. Preschoolers and older children enjoy assembling ingredients, measuring, mixing, and cutting under supervision.

While preschoolers and kindergartners are eager to work and learn, they're also easily distracted. Children in this age group usually need a lot of help to break jobs down into manageable parts. By age 7 or 8, however, children can harness their enthusiasm and focus on quite complicated tasks. Increasingly independent and cooperative, they like to be told that you appreciate their contribution to the family.

20 minutes earlier. At night, check that homework is finished and packed ready for school. Lay out clothes for the morning. Get the table ready for breakfast so all you have to add is food.

Not only did Paige find it hard to wake up in the morning, but the thought of food right away made her queasy. She felt ready to eat only after she had washed, dressed, fed the cat, and spent her first 10 minutes on the school bus catching up with developments in her friends' lives since the afternoon before. Her mother stopped trying to force the family breakfast on Paige. Instead, she packed a box of chilled milk or calcium-fortified orange juice and a granola bar in Paige's backpack. Sometimes she added a piece of fruit or cheese as well. That way, Paige could eat her breakfast on the bus and be ready for school by the end of the ride.

Some children really can't face eating first thing in the morning. If your child is one of them, try offering her a small glass of 100 percent fruit juice as soon as she wakes up. By the time she's dressed, she may be ready for breakfast.

It's not the end of the world if your child skips breakfast. Above all, it's not worth nagging your child or worrying unnecessarily and thus setting the scene for confrontations and upsets first thing in the morning. If your morning routine runs like clockwork, but your child still doesn't eat, pack a breakfast to eat on the bus or at snack time. She'll eat when she feels hungry. Emphasize cereals, low-fat dairy foods, and proteins, and keep the sugar and fat content moderate. Check the suggestions on page 61 for breakfast ideas.

School Menus: News from the Lunchroom

The big change with the school years is that many meals are eaten away from home. Most students have lunch at school, whether they eat cafeteria food or bring a bag lunch. Some children also have breakfast at school.

Many schools use the Food Guide Pyramid to teach the principles of good nutrition starting at the kindergarten level. Cafeterias usually provide sandwich- or salad-makings for those who don't want the dish of the day.

To stretch limited budgets, many schools contract with fast-food chains for lunches. School administrators can request changes in the standard dishes, however, to keep the fat content moderate. Chicken nuggets and fish sticks, for example, can be baked instead of fried; the salad bar should offer a selection of raw vegetables and low-fat dressings.

Most schools regularly send schedules of cafeteria menus home. With this advance information, you can plan on packing lunch on the days when the main course is one your child prefers not to eat.

School Lunches: You Can Make a Difference

Meal planning for schools is a complicated process. Menus have to allow for a wide range of tastes and restrictions. Budgets are limited. The foods that are available at lowest cost and require the least preparation are often high in fat, sugar,

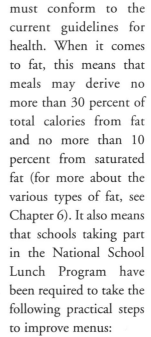

(MENU SUGGESTIONS)

BREAKFASTS TO GO

Dry cereal and yogurt
with berries or sliced fruit

Bagel or toasted English muffin
with peanut butter

Ham and low-fat cheese sandwich
on whole-wheat bread

Low-fat granola bar

Low-fat raisin-bran or fruit-oatmeal muffin

Warm cereal in an insulated container

Whole-wheat waffle spread with
"lite" cream cheese and strawberries

Whole-wheat banana-nut bread

100 percent fruit juice or low-fat milk;
insulated container of warm cocoa on
winter mornings

and sodium. According to the School Meals Initiative for Healthy Children set up in 1996, school lunch menus backed by federal subsidies must conform to the current guidelines for health. When it comes to fat, this means that meals may derive no more than 30 percent of total calories from fat and no more than 10 percent from saturated fat (for more about the various types of fat, see Chapter 6). It also means that schools taking part in the National School Lunch Program have been required to take the following practical steps to improve menus:

- Adding more fruits, vegetables, and grains to menus.
- Balancing menus by using foods from each of the five groups.
- Reducing overall fat content by serving more vegetarian main courses, less beef and pork, and fewer fried foods.
- Varying menus by serving more ethnic dishes, such as pasta and tacos.

To back up efforts at the lunchroom level, the U.S. Department of Agriculture set up Team Nutrition, a program to improve children's eating habits and raise their awareness about the links between food and health. Participation in the program is voluntary, but within 3 years of its start-up in 1995, Team Nutrition had supplied curriculum guides and classroom kits to 20,000 public and private schools across the country.

There's also a push at the state and local levels to help children eat better. In many communities, children at grade-school level are learning not only how to cook food but also how to grow a variety of produce. Courses combine food production and preparation with valuable lessons about history, economics, social science, and math.

If you're not satisfied with the choices available in your child's school cafeteria, get involved in the PTA and brainstorm some healthful alternatives, as parents and teachers all over the country are doing. In a small town in upstate New York, for example, children at the only elementary school expanded their social studies project on India to include making vegetable curry with a spice mixture they had ground themselves. They learned to cook and enjoy many of the healthful grains and legumes—lentils, chickpeas, bulgur wheat, brown rice, and beans—that are staples of Indian cooking but not often seen in school lunches. As a change of pace, the children celebrated Martin Luther King Day by combining black-eyed peas, corn, and collards in a soul-food stew. Their enthusiasm led the local supermarket to stock grains and greens that brought about a mini-revolution in the community's diet.

In West Virginia, a state-sponsored booklet shows teachers how to introduce children to foods from around the world in social studies classes. The booklet includes recipes that can be adapted to classroom and school cafeteria use. Oregon schoolchildren as young as 5 were consulted on what should be served in school lunches. The result was a surge in children's consumption of fruits and vegetables.

Even if you haven't the time or resources to revamp the school cafeteria, you may be able to see that the salad bar offers a good selection of raw vegetables and low-fat dressings. Vending machine choices can also be modified to eliminate high-fat and empty-calorie munchies and

▷ HEALTHY CHOICES FOR VENDING MACHINES

INSTEAD OF	SUGGEST
Potato chips	Baked tortilla chips
Artificially flavored and colored corn and cheese snacks	Popcorn
Candy bars	Granola bars; trail mix
Sweetened, fruit-flavored roll-ups	Fruits, dried or fresh
Fruit-flavored drinks with added sugar; soda pop	Water; unsweetened 100 percent fruit juices
Whole milk; full-fat yogurt	Skim or low-fat milk; yogurt
Ice cream	Sherbet; Italian ice; pure fruit popsicles; frozen yogurt
Creme-filled sandwich cookies; chocolate-chip cookies	Fig bar cookies; graham crackers

provide healthy snacks that include more fresh fruit and low-fat dairy products, as well as water and 100 percent fruit juice instead of sodas.

Try to get your child's school to stock healthy choices in the vending machines.

"But All the Other Kids Have Candy"
Packing bag lunches gives you lots of opportunities to develop your own creative ideas based on the Food Guide Pyramid. It's also a good time to get children actively involved in nutrition by planning a balanced meal and helping to prepare it. When children help prepare food, they'll often eat dishes their parents wouldn't dream they'd like.

Many schools forbid lunch-box trading, which cuts the risk that your child will trade his fresh fruit dessert for someone else's candy. Sooner or later, however, you're going to hear, "*All* the other kids get candy in their lunch boxes!" or "It's not fair: Why do I always get carrots and fruit when everybody else gets potato chips and cookies?"

You can repeat the message, "Because those other choices aren't good, even though they don't do any harm once in a while." And there are other ways. Children at the elementary school level love to show off their learning. Ask your child to teach you what he's learned at school about the Food Guide Pyramid, then pool what you know and come up with some joint guidelines for healthful choices. Even kindergartners are old enough to understand why fresh fruits and vegetables are better than chips and cookies, or why candy and soda are okay as occasional treats but not as lunch-box staples. So that your child won't feel deprived, you could let him mark the calendar with a weekly "treat day." On other days, his lunch box might include nonfat oatmeal-raisin or fig bar cookies for dessert, or a bag of baked tortilla chips with salsa for dipping.

 TAKE LESSONS FROM HOME TO SCHOOL

At home, give children the job of preparing the salads for family meals. Even children too young to handle a sharp knife can tear up lettuce and other greens, then toss them with just enough dressing to make the ingredients shiny without leaving a puddle in the bottom of the bowl. Suggest that your child prepare his or her own salads at the salad bar in the school cafeteria.

Clean Hands, Healthy Eating
When you pack a bag lunch, thoroughly wash and dry all reusable containers, and wash your hands just as you do before preparing any other meal (also see Chapter 13). Remember that the lunch is going to sit unrefrigerated in a backpack or locker for several hours. Choose sandwich fillings that don't need to be refrigerated and avoid meats or salads that may spoil. Pack crushable foods in plastic containers. Wash fruit well. Peel and wash vegetables such as carrots and wrap them in plastic or wax paper. Always discard partly consumed drinks and foods such as yogurt.

It's a good idea to invest in an insulated soft-pack and an unbreakable insulated drink bottle. If you haven't got a cold pack, get into the routine of freezing juice boxes and plastic bottles of water. Tucked into the bag, the drink is thawed by lunchtime and helps to keep other foods cool.

After-School Snacks
Keep your kitchen stocked with healthy snack foods such as fresh fruits, raw vegetables with dips, baked tortillas and salsa, whole-grain crack-

▷ **H₂O + SUGAR + FOOD DYE + BOTTLE = $$$**

The sports drinks youngsters see advertised aren't necessary; at the same time, they won't do any harm. Water, however, is a much less expensive way to keep tissues hydrated and systems working. For extra zing, add a few slices of lemon or lime.

ers, pretzels, and low-fat yogurt to fill in after-school gaps. This is especially important when both parents work outside the home and children are in charge of their own after-school snacks and sometimes dinner as well. Avoid having a supply of cookies, cakes, ice cream, and fatty, salty snack foods on hand. Children who have unsupervised access to such foods can gain unwanted weight. However, served as occasional treats, these foods do no harm and provide variety.

School-Age Children and Sports

Children at grade school level should be getting plenty of exercise and taking part in organized sports where there are opportunities to do so. School-age athletes can get all the nutrition they need from the recommended servings of the Food Guide Pyramid, although you may have to increase portion sizes or add a snack or two for very active children. A young athlete will feel most comfortable when performing if she eats a low-fat, high-carbohydrate meal, such as pasta with tomato-vegetable sauce, several hours before an event. High-performance supplements and weight-training programs to reduce body fat or increase muscle mass have no place in school athletics. They won't improve athletic performance and may be harmful.

Keep the Water Flowing

Apart from a balanced diet with enough calories for energy and growth, active children need plenty of water. School-age athletes are especially vulnerable to dehydration when playing in hot, humid weather. Parents and coaches should keep a close watch to make sure that children drink plenty of water before and during practices and games, even though they may not feel thirsty. Thirst lags behind water losses, and by the time children feel thirsty, they may already be dehydrated. A school-age child should drink the equivalent of six to eight glasses of water daily, and more during exercise or in hot weather. Remember, young children have a harder time coping with extremes of temperature than adolescents and adults.

Children and Constipation

Constipation is one of the most over-reported and least understood symptoms. People have the idea that constipation means not having a daily bowel movement. They think youngsters will get sick if they don't have a movement every day. Not so. Many children (and adults) have several bowel movements every day, while others go 2 or 3 days or even longer, then pass a stool of normal consistency. A person is constipated only when the stool is hard or dry and can't be passed without straining or causing pain. Constipation may occur when the diet lacks fiber or fluid. It's also fairly common after a viral illness, when children may not drink enough and are less active than usual.

To keep your children's bowel movements normal, make sure they eat high-fiber foods such as fruits, vegetables, and whole-grain breads and cereals. Nutrition experts recommend as a general rule that a person's daily intake of fiber should equal his or her age plus 5 grams (thus, for a 7-year-old, 7 + 5 = 12 grams a day) up to a maximum of 35 grams a day. Oat bran cereal and pop-corn are good sources of fiber that many young people like to eat. A couple of prunes or a small glass of prune juice can help stimulate bowel function. Prunes contain a natural laxative, called isatin, as well as lots of soluble fiber and sorbitol—a naturally occurring, nonabsorbable sugar alcohol—both of which have laxative effects. Apple juice and pear juice are also good sources of sorbitol; however, cooked apples, such as in applesauce, may contribute to constipation and are often given to help children with diarrhea. Plenty of water—6 to 8 glasses a day—is needed to augment water in the stool and help keep bowel movements regular. (Also see Chapter 7.)

"He Doesn't Eat, No Matter What I Say"

There are school-age children who seem to eat next to nothing. They have little appetite or may not enjoy eating. To their parents' amazement, these children keep on growing, which shows that they're getting enough to eat. Some of these children feel uncomfortable if they try to conform to the usual daily pattern of three relatively large meals. They are happier nibbling on several small meals over the course of the day.

Coaxing a nibbler to eat larger, less frequent meals isn't helpful. In fact, studies show that children consume less when parents try to persuade them to eat. Some nibblers are also put off when parents praise them for eating. To these children, attention to eating makes them feel as if they're being forced to eat. On the other hand, it isn't a good idea to leave food out for unrestricted snacking. It leads to bad habits of constant picking and the food may spoil.

Let your nibbler eat as much as he wants at the three meals and additional snacks you serve each day. He may eat less at mealtimes and more at snacktimes than other members of the family. At least you'll be sure that he's getting the amount and variety he needs while the family meal schedule is maintained.

Feeding Difficulties and Picky Eaters

Children's food preferences veer all over the menu: Today they want third helpings of spinach, tomorrow they *never* eat anything green. Trying as it can be to keep up with the whims of an easygoing child, the picky eater presents a challenge of a different order. Some picky eaters are difficult feeders from the beginning. For them, picky eating and faddishness are part of a progression from fussiness and colic to extreme resistance to new foods. Some children are picky because they are unusually sensitive to certain tastes and textures, while others use food as a tool to manipulate their parents and gain attention.

Appetite and hunger are two different things. Hunger is the body's signal that it needs fuel. By contrast, appetite is a learned behavior involving pleasure and other emotions associated with eating. Hunger is present from birth; appetite develops over time. Children learn positive and negative attitudes to eating from observing what goes on around them. For example, a child who takes part in relaxed family meals from his early months is more likely to look forward to eating than one who's never allowed to leave the table until he has finished everything on his plate. When parents use food as a bribe or reward ("You'll get double dessert if you clean your plate!"), children quickly learn that they can use food in a similar way, and may try to manipulate their parents by eating or refusing meals. Parents worried by their daughter's refusal to eat may be surprised to learn that the child is only following her mother's example of nonstop dieting.

Many problems related to picky eating gradually disappear after a child begins eating regularly away from parental supervision. For example, children in group childcare tend to copy the way their friends eat. A picky older child may eat school lunches without a fuss, although he continues his picky behavior at meals he shares with his parents. Finally, many faddish eaters get more pleasure from attention-seeking than they do from feeding. Therefore, while it's acceptable to compliment satisfactory behavior at the end of the meal, food refusals and demands for attention should be ignored or managed by promptly terminating the meal. If you've come to expect pickiness as part of your family's mealtime routine, it may be advisable to seek outside help, starting with your pediatrician. (For problems related to eating disorders, see Chapter 10.)

Some children fail to develop pleasure in eating because medical problems or treatments interfere with the normal feeding process. For example, a child who had to be fed by tube for a long period because she was premature or sick as a newborn may dislike the sensation of food in her mouth. Children with persistent nasal congestion, a frequent complication of tube feeding or allergies,

FOOD PROBLEMS THAT CROP UP DURING THE SCHOOL YEARS

When my child stays over at friends' houses, he eats all kinds of junk foods that I never serve at home. Should I be concerned?
An occasional meal or snack including junk foods isn't going to harm your child if his normal diet at home is healthy. (See p. 54.)

My child is much smaller than all her classmates. She's growing steadily but very slowly. Should she eat more?
Each child grows at his or her own rate, depending on thousands of inherited and environmental influences. There aren't any hard-and-fast rules about how many calories a school-age child needs to eat. As long as your child is eating a variety of foods and is gaining in height and weight, there's no cause for concern. In fact, trying to make her eat more may have the opposite effect from what you intend. (Also see pp. 59 and 65.)

My child doesn't feel like eating right after she gets up. Is breakfast such a big deal at this age?
Breakfast is important. Children who don't eat breakfast may have trouble staying alert. Revise your child's morning schedule to allow more time. Waking her with a

have a reduced sense of taste and smell and, therefore, take little pleasure in eating. Nowadays, children who require special feeding techniques, such as tubes, are given appropriate oral stimulation—so-called sham feeding—to help them adapt to feeding by mouth. If your child has feeding difficulties related to medical problems or treatments, your pediatrician will advise you about where to find appropriate resources for help and support.

In studying how children respond to efforts to get them to eat, researchers have agreed on a few universal truths:

FIRST: It is the parents' responsibility to provide the food, and it's the child's decision to eat it.

SECOND: Bribes and coercion are counterproductive. They make children resistant to foods they feel neutral about, and make them actively dislike foods to which they're indifferent. The child may well reason: "If they have to bribe me to eat this stuff, it must be bad."

THIRD: Mealtimes are for eating and socializing, not for playing games. Make meals a time for enjoyable family interaction in which children want to take part.

FOURTH: Meals should be kept to a reasonable time-limit in keeping with the child's attention span.

glass of 100 percent fruit juice may be helpful. Or try packing a brown-bag breakfast to eat on the way to school. (For more about children and breakfast, see p. 59.)

My child refuses to eat in the school cafeteria, and when I look at the menus, I can see why. Aren't there any guidelines for school lunches?

School lunches backed with federal funds must conform to current health standards. For example, meals may have only 30 percent of total calories from fat and no more than 10 percent from saturated fat. There are lots of exciting, healthy developments in school lunch programs. (Read about them starting on p. 60.)

My son is really into sports. He says he could improve his performance by taking vitamin and mineral supplements. Since these products are not drugs, is there any harm in letting him try them?

Nutritional supplements won't help performance, and some can actually be harmful. School-age athletes get all the nutrition they need from a normal, balanced diet. (Read about school-age children and sports on p. 64.)

CHAPTER 5

The Adolescent Years

Sheila Wilder was torn between pride and exasperation over her teenage daughter, Marissa. On the one hand, Sheila was overjoyed when Marissa was selected to represent her high school in the regional gymnastics championships. On the other, she felt angry when Marissa picked at meals and didn't eat enough, Sheila thought, for a still developing teenager involved in school and social activities, as well as hours of daily practice.

Marissa seemed to be overconcerned with her weight, insisting that she looked fat in her leotard despite her mother's reassurances. In an effort to shed this invisible fat, Marissa refused milk and dairy products ("too much fat"), meat ("gross"), and many breads and cereals ("too starchy"). She accused her mother of interfering when Sheila tried to persuade her to eat a more balanced diet. The best course, Sheila decided, was to seek impartial advice before the tension grew unbearable or Marissa developed health problems.

Listening to the pediatrician who had looked after her since kindergarten, Marissa remained unconvinced. However, she agreed to try some of his recommendations. Accepting the importance of calcium for bone strength, Marissa promised to eat a helping of nonfat yogurt every morning and to pour skim milk on her cereal. Her pediatrician also suggested a daily dose of an over-the-counter calcium-based antacid, to make sure Marissa got enough calcium. The doctor gave her, in writing, a low-fat diet plan that included grains and legumes (rather than the meat she disliked) for protein and iron, as well as plenty of vegetables and fruit for vitamins and fiber. Marissa also said she would try to weigh herself no more than once a week, instead of every night and morning, as she had been doing.

At the peak of the growth spurt, an adolescent may easily grow 4 inches in a year. This increase in height parallels the changes taking place within the body. The heart, for example, doubles in size, as does the lung capacity. Similar changes take place in nearly all other organs.

The pediatrician scheduled a series of follow-up visits to monitor Marissa's progress. He found her weight to be within the normal range for her height. Finally, he explained to Marissa and Sheila that if he noticed signs that the teenager wasn't keeping her pledges, he would refer her promptly to a program to prevent the development of an eating disorder. For her part, Sheila was relieved that Marissa had agreed to be responsible for her own eating behavior and that her pediatrician was going to follow her regularly.

How They Grow

The rate of growth picks up a bit before children develop the first signs of sexual maturation—breast budding in girls and growth of the testes in boys—then accelerates rapidly. Growth reaches a peak at about age 12 in girls, before menstruation begins. In boys, the peak rate occurs later, at about age 14. These numbers are just averages, however; for individual youngsters, sexual maturation and increased growth may begin as much as 2 years earlier or 2 years later.

Until puberty, boys and girls the same age are similar in size. With the onset of puberty, but before the first menstrual period (menarche), girls have reached their growth peak and are looking down on their male classmates from a lofty advantage of $1^1/2$ inches. Although boys start puberty later, they soon overtake girls. By age 14, boys equal girls in height and, after growth is complete, are 5 inches taller, on average, than girls.

Where Energy Goes

It takes measurable energy to carry out the various vital functions and keep the body healthy. This is called the resting metabolic rate. Adolescents also need calories to fuel their physical activity. On a daily basis, normally active teenagers use up one third to one half of all the calories they consume in physical activity. Of course, the amount of energy used for physical activity by individual teenagers varies—from less than half the energy in a sedentary adolescent's diet to much more than half for a high-performing athlete. Finally, teenagers need a small number of additional calories to power the adolescent growth spurt. An adequate energy supply is essential for this process.

During adolescence, young people become increasingly independent of their families, although a good deal of this so-called independence actually consists of doing exactly what their friends are doing. A teenager would rather join a group of friends for fast food—if that's what the group is doing—than make polite conversation around the family table. Furthermore, a typical teenager's schedule—crowded with school and extracurricular activities, sports, perhaps a part-time job, sleeping late, and time spent just hanging out with friends—may not leave a lot of time to join the family at meals. For these and other reasons, many adolescents seem to eat most of their meals on the run. However, even if your teenager is eating out more often than in, you can encourage her to get balanced nutrition with low-fat, healthful choices based on the Food Guide Pyramid (see p. 90).

Learning to Deal with Outside Pressure

Because teenagers watch many hours of television, their food choices tend to be heavily influenced by advertising. A commercial may suggest, for instance, that eating certain snacks or drinking the "right" soda will help teenagers fit in with the group and have a good time. Often clever and memorable, ads are designed to sell products, not to instruct adolescents about healthy eating. Advice about nutrition offered in teenage magazines is generally sound. In some cases, though, it may be influenced by advertisers and often focuses on dieting or building muscle.

As your child enters adolescence, continue to deliver the message that ads are designed for one purpose: to manipulate consumers. Urge your teenager to read between the lines of advertisements and commercials, and to read the labels on

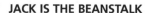

JACK IS THE BEANSTALK

The hands and feet get bigger first. Then the legs grow longer, giving the typical gangly, coltish look of the early teenage years. Soon the jaw begins to lengthen and the facial features enlarge. Because different parts of the body grow at different rates, a youngster may look as if he's nothing but elbows and knees one month and all ears and nose the next. Finally, the trunk and chest catch up, and all the parts of the puzzle fit into place.

EATING PATTERNS CHANGE

Eating together has been a way to strengthen family ties throughout every age and culture. Young people entering adolescence usually have fairly well-established habits and preferences based on their families' approaches to food. However, as adolescents grow older, they eat fewer meals with their families. The way their friends eat may become the dominant influence on eating patterns.

food products to find out what the ads don't admit. (Read more about dealing with outside influences in Chapter 11.)

What Are Adolescents Really Eating?

Schools teach children about nutrition, often starting with a Food Guide Pyramid in the classroom as early as kindergarten. The healthy message continues on up through the grades, stressing the importance of vegetables and fruits (five or more a day, as advised by the USDA Food Guide Pyramid, the American Heart Association, the National Cancer Institute, and others); complex carbohydrates, such as grains and cereals; low-fat dairy and protein choices; and fiber. With new government guidelines, many school lunch programs have switched to more healthful and varied menus. Yet surveys show poor eating patterns that may have adverse effects on the future health.

Researchers who compared adolescents' food intakes with the Food Guide Pyramid recommendations (also see Chapter 6) found that on the

FAST FOODS CAN BE HEALTHY FOODS

Many of the fast-food restaurants where teenagers like to gather offer a selection of healthy alternatives:

- A chicken fajita instead of a breaded chicken sandwich.

- A "lean" burger instead of an outsize special with lots of fat-laden trimmings.

- A baked potato instead of high-fat French fries.

- A main-course salad from the salad bar with low-fat dressing.

- Nonfat frozen yogurt with a fresh fruit topping instead of ice cream or a wedge of pie.

- Water or a low-fat milkshake instead of soda or a regular shake.

Teenagers will eat pizza even when they turn down almost any other food. Luckily, pizza can be a well-balanced and nutritious meal—a healthy balance of complex carbohydrates, vegetables, protein, and a little fat—if it's garnished with vegetables such as tomato sauce, mushrooms, eggplant, and peppers instead of high-fat toppings such as sausage, pepperoni, and extra cheese.

whole, teenage boys ate a much healthier diet than girls the same age. For example, boys met at least the minimum recommendations for grains, vegetables, and meat, though their choices tended to be high in fat. By contrast, adolescent girls failed to achieve the minimum in any food group. As they grew older, both boys and girls ate more vegetables and meat, although the increase in vegetables was offset by a corresponding decrease in fruit

▷ CALORIES TO GROW ON

Energy resources available to the child's developing body are used, first, for vital functions and, second, for physical activity. What's left over goes to growth and sexual maturation. If the energy supply is lacking, growth suffers. But even at the height of the adolescent growth spurt, a teenager uses only about 100 calories a day—equivalent to the energy in two slices of bread—to grow.

consumption. However, nearly a quarter of the vegetables the youngsters counted as daily servings were French fries, which are high in fat and have limited nutritional value. The intake of dark green and deep yellow vegetables was very low compared with recommended levels.

Particularly disturbing was the low level of dairy food consumption among teenage girls. Only about one girl in five was eating the recommended two or three daily servings of dairy foods, and consumption of the grain and fruit groups was not much better. Intake of vegetables and meat was healthier, but still far below the levels recommended in the Food Guide Pyramid. The

researchers suggested that the low energy (calorie) intake among teenage girls reflected the typical overriding concern with weight in this age group.

The researchers warned that adolescents who met none of the recommended intakes were getting far less than the Recommended Dietary Allowances (RDAs) for essential vitamins and minerals, including vitamin B_6, folic acid, calcium, iron, and zinc, and their diets had far too little fiber. Invariably, teenagers who failed to meet the minimum in any food group were eating high levels of added sugars. In all age groups, children consumed more fat than the recommended quantity (no more than 30 percent of calories); they obtained 40 percent of their energy from fats and added sugars without meeting the Food Guide Pyramid recommendations for grains, fruit, and low-fat dairy foods. Even though teenage boys weren't eating according to the Food Guide Pyramid, they still had the healthiest diet, whereas teenage girls and children from minority and low-income households had the least healthy patterns of eating. These adolescent eating habits differ from the prevalent pattern among adults, where only about 9 percent fail to meet the minimum recommendations in any food group.

Adolescents are often quite knowledgeable about calories, fat, and cholesterol. However, apart from school courses in nutrition, many tend to get nutritional information from television programs and talk shows. Such programs are prone to deliver endless, sensational stories about instant weight-loss programs and diet supplements "guaranteed" to burn off fat. What's worrisome is that these young people may skip meals in favor of snacks or convenience food eaten while watching television. For some middle-class and even affluent teenagers, the family dinner table may be something they see only in TV situation comedies.

CARBOHYDRATES AND CALORIES IN A FEW EVERYDAY FOODS

Food	Carbohydrates (grams)	Calories
Breads, cereals		
White or whole wheat, 1 slice	12	65
Bagel (1 medium)	38	200
Corn flakes, sugar-frosted, ¾ cup	26	110
Cracker, graham, 2 pieces	11	60
English muffin	27	140
Taco shell	7	50
Toaster pastry, 1	35	195
Fruits, juices		
Apple, 1 medium	21	80
Banana, 1 medium	27	105
Orange juice, fresh, ½ cup	13	55
Raisins, 1½-ounce package	10	40
Pasta, cooked firm, drained (1 cup)		
Macaroni	39	190
Egg noodles	37	200
Spaghetti	39	190
Rice (1 cup)		
Brown or enriched white	25	115
Vegetables and legumes		
Black beans, cooked, ½ cup	20	115
Black-eyed peas, cooked, ½ cup	18	95
Carrot, raw, 1 medium	7	30
Celery, raw, 1 stalk	1	5
Corn, boiled, 1 ear	19	85
Kidney beans, cooked, ½ cup	20	110
Potato, baked, 1 medium	50	220
Potato, French-fried in vegetable oil, frozen (10 pieces)	20	160
Yogurt, low-fat, 8 ounces		
Plain	16	145
Fruit-flavored	43	230

It's hard to convince teenagers of the importance of good nutrition for their future years, to prevent cancer, heart disease, and other serious illnesses. However, teenage athletes may accept the importance of eating well to improve performance. All adolescents want to be physically attractive (even though their notions of what constitutes attractiveness may differ from yours) and may adapt their diets to achieve this goal. Girls and boys alike should be encouraged to develop an interest in food, healthy eating, and exercise to stay slim and fit.

How Many Calories?

As a general rule, moderately active adolescent boys should consume about 2,700 calories a day, and girls need about 2,300 calories. It's impossible to specify an exact number of calories because individual energy needs depend on size and build, growth rate, and level of physical activity. A rapidly developing boy who is involved in a challenging athletics program, for example, may burn up 5,000 calories or even more a day, whereas a girl who tends to be sedentary might need only about 2,000 calories. In adolescence, as in the early school years, the best guide is a satisfactory rate of growth—if the young person is still growing—along with good levels of energy and fitness.

Where Those Calories Come From

Complex carbohydrates—starchy foods such as pasta, breads, cereals, rice, beans, lentils, and other legumes—are the bedrock of a healthful diet. Adolescents, like adults, should get 55 to 60 percent of their daily calories from carbohydrates. This amount allows for a large proportion of complex carbohydrates and a smaller amount of simple carbohydrates, or sugars, including the naturally occurring sugars in fruits and vegetables. Only 30 percent of calories, at most, should come from fats, with no more than one third of this allowance (that is, 10 percent of total daily calories) from saturated fat—the kind that tends to stay solid at room temperature. (Most of the fat in meat and dairy products is saturated.) Finally, although protein is important, it should not make up more than 10 to 12 percent of the calories consumed.

How Big Is a Serving?

Serving sizes for teenagers are the same as for adults. (For more about the recommended daily servings, check out the Food Guide Pyramid on p. 90.)

The Iron Age

A teenager's blood volume expands to keep up with the body's increasing need for oxygen, which is carried by iron-rich hemoglobin in the red blood cells. The RDA of iron for adolescent girls is 15 milligrams a day, and some experts recommend up to 30 milligrams for girls who are heavily involved in athletics. The RDA for teenage boys is 12 milligrams of iron a day. (Also see What Makes Sammy [and Samantha] Run? p. 79.)

Lack of iron means lower levels of hemoglobin leading to anemia, tiredness, weakness, increased susceptibility to infection, and other symptoms. Most people are aware that iron is important in adolescent girls' diets to make up for losses in menstrual blood. Our bodies retrieve iron from old blood cells. Therefore, boys and men don't need to consume as much iron as girls and women, who lose iron during their menstrual period. However, although boys generally have higher hemoglobin levels than girls, boys also can develop iron deficiency; they need plenty of iron

Bread	1 slice	
Cereal, dry	1 ounce (3/4 cup)*	
Cereal, cooked	1 ounce (1/2 cup)	
Pasta, rice (cooked)	1 ounce (1/2 cup)	
Vegetables (cooked)	1/2 cup	
Fruit	1 medium piece, e.g., 1 apple or pear	
Milk, yogurt	1 cup	
Cheese	11/2 ounces (11/2-inch cube or 2 precut slices)	
Meat, poultry, fish	2 to 3 ounces (about the size of a deck of playing cards)	

*All cup measures are a standard 8-ounce measuring cup.

in the diet. A boy or girl may be iron deficient without actually being anemic. Athletes taking part in strenuous sports during the growth spurt have a special need for dietary iron to offset iron losses in the digestive tract, urine, and sweat.

There are two different types of dietary iron. Heme iron is found in foods of animal origin, such as meat, fish and shellfish, and poultry. Nonheme iron occurs in plants; good sources are dark green leafy vegetables and dried fruits. Iron-fortified breads and cereals are also important sources of the mineral.

Our bodies absorb only between 5 and 20 percent of the iron we eat, depending on the composition of the meal. With heme iron, about 20 percent is absorbed no matter how it's prepared and served. Nonheme iron is less easily absorbed, but we can increase the absorption rate by eating sources of nonheme iron—such as legumes and fortified breads and grains—together with foods that contain some heme iron, or foods rich in vitamin C. These include citrus fruits and vegeta-

bles such as cauliflower, broccoli, tomatoes, and potatoes. Meat contains a substance that is also known to promote nonheme iron absorption, although it has not yet been isolated and identified. Combining a small amount of meat, therefore, with iron-rich legumes or beans can boost the amount of iron that is absorbed.

Tannins, phytates, and calcium in foods such as tea, bran, and milk, respectively, can hinder the absorption of nonheme iron eaten at the same meal by as much as 50 percent. If your child has been diagnosed with iron-deficiency anemia, or if you're otherwise concerned about her iron intake, see that she drinks tea and milk only at snacktimes. At mealtimes, serve fruits and vegetables rich in vitamin C or a glass of citrus juice, to help her absorb more iron.

Lean meat, poultry, and fish are good sources of iron. Other sources include soy products such as tofu, chickpeas (garbanzo beans), lentils, and white beans. If you cook an acidic food, such as tomato sauce or chili, in a cast-iron pot, some of the min-

With the twin goals of helping adolescents develop their peak bone mass and preventing osteoporosis in older adults, in 1997 the National Academy of Sciences issued the following new recommendations for an adequate daily intake of calcium.

Age group (years)	Adequate intake (milligrams per day)
1–3	500
4–8	800
9–18	1,300
19–50	1,000
51–70	1,200
71+	1,200

eral is leached out into the food and can supply a little dietary iron; however, some vitamins may be lost.

Growing Bones

A good supply of calcium is essential during adolescence. Growing children build up approximately 40 to 45 percent of their peak adult bone mass during the teenage years, and calcium is the main building block of bone. The National Academy of Sciences recommends 1,300 milligrams a day as an adequate intake of calcium for adolescents (see box, left). A teenager should easily be able to reach this level with four daily servings from the milk, yogurt, and cheese group plus a good intake of green vegetables. Milk and dairy products made from fortified milk may be the best source, because they also contain vitamin D, which promotes the absorption of calcium.

▷ STRONG BONES NOW, STRONG BONES LATER

Most of the calcium in the bones is laid down during adolescence and early adulthood. After that time, calcium in the bones can be turned over or lost, but not added. Therefore, a good intake of calcium during adolescence is crucial for reducing the risk of osteoporosis and disabling fractures later in life.

After about age 30, bone mass declines steadily in both women and men, and the rate of loss accelerates sharply in women once they reach menopause. The greater the peak bone mass at early adulthood, the less the risk of osteoporosis—or weakened bones—is later in life.

Women are at greater risk than men for developing osteoporosis, and women of Northern European and Asian ancestry are at higher risk than those of African and Mediterranean descent. Many other factors appear to be involved, including smoking and having a slender build, fair skin, and family history of the disease. All women, irrespective of their risk factor profile, should try to keep their bones healthy with adequate intakes of calcium and vitamin D, and regular, moderate, weight-bearing exercise.

Many teenagers, particularly weight-conscious girls, shun calcium-rich dairy products because they're afraid of getting fat, but low-fat and non-fat milk products are widely available. Removing fat doesn't take away calcium, and reduced-fat dairy products are just as rich in calcium as the full-fat versions.

Tofu is also an excellent source of calcium. Dark green leafy vegetables, such as kale and turnip greens, are low in calories and have as much calcium, ounce for ounce, as dairy foods. Calcium-fortified orange juice is a good choice because the vitamin C in the juice promotes the absorption of calcium. Vitamin D is also needed to absorb calcium. The body can make vitamin D when the skin is exposed to the sun. Dietary sources include fortified milk, eggs, and butter. For adolescent girls who won't drink milk and don't eat enough calcium, many pediatricians suggest a daily dose of calcium-containing antacid tablets, which are available without prescription.

Folate

All teenagers should consume plenty of leafy green vegetables, fruits, and fortified cereals for folate (also called folic acid), a vitamin our bodies need to make the DNA and RNA in cells, as well as for the formation of healthy red blood cells. Low levels of folate in pregnant women are known to cause serious birth defects involving babies' spines and nervous systems. Therefore, folate is particularly important for adolescent girls and young women, to make sure that they will have adequate levels when they eventually prepare for pregnancy.

Fiber

Teenagers should aim for the recommended five servings a day of vegetables and fruits, to give them

▷ PHOSPHORUS

Phosphorus is another mineral needed for bone formation. The RDA for phosphorus is 1,200 milligrams a day for 9- to 18-year-olds. Phosphorus is found in most protein-rich foods, such as meat, eggs, and legumes, and generally occurs also in the same foods as calcium. In fact, phosphorus is so abundant that most people routinely consume more of it than of calcium. Also, our bodies absorb phosphorus more easily than calcium—about 70 percent of a given quantity of phosphorus compared with 30 to 40 percent of calcium.

adequate amounts of vitamins A, C, and E, and other cancer-fighting phytochemicals, and to supply fiber to keep things moving. A regular intake of fiber may help prevent many disorders, including cancer and heart disease, in middle age and later.

Exercise and Healthy Bones

Physical activity—especially strength training and weight-bearing exercise—is good for bone. Combined with a balanced diet, physical activity not only strengthens bone, but also stimulates the production of hormones that protect bones, and generates electrical activity within the bones that promotes growth and repair. Exercise also boosts the flow of blood and nutrients to the bones.

Although weight-bearing exercise helps strengthen bones, some girls exercise and/or diet so much that they lack the body fat needed to produce hormones essential for bone formation.

Other girls avoid milk—an important source of bone-building calcium—because they think it will make them fat. In all cases, these girls are susceptible to osteoporosis. Serious effects on bone formation may appear before such women reach age 40.

It is crucial that adolescent girls pay special attention to their need for calcium and vitamin D. Sports coaches and ballet teachers, as well as parents, have a responsibility to help girl athletes and young performers eat a healthful, balanced diet. Typical teenagers find it hard to picture themselves in middle age and beyond. Thus, preaching a diet for tomorrow's health may not be persuasive. It's better to emphasize the importance of good nutrition—including plenty of calcium—to achieve the best performance today.

Zinc

Zinc—found in meat, fish, poultry, and dairy products, as well as shellfish, whole grains, dried beans, and nuts—is necessary for many metabolic processes as well as for wound healing and sexual maturation. The RDA for zinc is 15 milligrams a day for adolescents. A high intake of iron and calcium may slightly decrease zinc absorption. However, zinc is easily absorbed in the presence of protein. At all ages, our bodies need zinc and iron in similar amounts.

Other Essential Minerals

Trace minerals needed to keep enzyme systems and metabolic processes functioning properly include copper, selenium, iodine, chromium, manganese, and molybdenum. A balanced diet provides the

▷ ANABOLIC STEROIDS AND OTHER PERFORMANCE ENHANCERS

Athletes may be tempted to use supplements to improve athletic performance. Expensive nutritional products such as power bars and shakes are popular, but haven't been shown to enhance performance. Amino acid preparations, such as arginine and ornithine, have no proven value; one product, tryptophan, was banned by the FDA because of serious toxicity. No studies have evaluated the effects of creatine supplements on the growth, development, or health of children and adolescents.

Anabolic steroids can stimulate muscle development, but are both dangerous to health and illegal. In boys, these synthetic male hormones can damage the testicles, cause the breasts to grow, and stunt growth. In girls, anabolic steroids cause a masculine appearance, including abnormal development of the sexual organs. Steroids alter the blood cholesterol levels and may increase the risk of heart disease in both males and females. They can have profound effects on the personality. Long-term use has been associated with severe liver disease, including cancer.

Although the adverse effects are widely known, anabolic steroids are still distributed illegally among adolescents in middle school and high school. Make sure your teenagers are aware of the dangers associated with these and other illicit drugs. Show them alternative, healthy ways of building strength and gaining an edge on the competition.

MASTER OF THE UNIVERSE IN THREE EASY STAGES

Boys' growth follows a distinct three-part sequence that's tied directly to the rate of sexual maturation, not to height. First, a boy rapidly grows taller. Then, about a year after his growth has peaked, he starts to develop muscle mass. By this time, his beard and chest hair have started to grow. Finally, he develops strength and endurance. A scrawny, late-maturing kid won't turn into a master of the universe by taking nutritional supplements.

Attempting strenuous strength training too soon can overstress the musculoskeletal system. After a boy has reached the right stage of development, he should be able to gain muscle by keeping to a well-planned and supervised strength-training program and diet. He should aim to increase his weight by no more than one pound a week.

RDA or—if the RDA is not yet known—the recognized safe level of every known vitamin and mineral. Only in unusual cases, when a child has a chronic condition or special dietary needs, do pediatricians prescribe supplements. Vitamin and mineral supplements offer no benefit, are costly and, when taken to excess, can be harmful.

What Makes Sammy (and Samantha) Run?
Scott, at age 15, was only beginning to show physical changes that most of his classmates had long since experienced. Self-conscious about his smaller size and relative lack of development, Scott was tempted to start a diet and work-out program he had read about in a body-building magazine. He asked his high school athletics director to recommend a protein supplement.

"Don't waste your money," the coach told Scott. "Lots of guys think supplements will help them bulk up and mature faster. Believe me, they don't help and they could hurt you.

"Eat a regular diet and keep exercising. You have a good chance of making the swim team if you work at it."

Teenage athletes are prepared to work hard and train for hours at a time, but many are also susceptible to the notion that there is a magic formula for gaining a competitive edge. The formula generally involves manipulating the diet.

There's no nutritional magic trick for improving athletic prowess. A balanced intake from the five basic food groups (check the Food Guide Pyramid, p. 90) should provide the nutrients a young athlete needs for growth and performance. At a minimum, the daily intake should include:

- Six servings from the breads and cereals group
- Two servings from the meat/protein group.
- Five servings from the vegetables and fruits groups.
- Four servings from the dairy group.

Carbohydrates for Energy
About 50 to 55 percent of an athlete's daily energy requirement should come from carbohydrates, as recommended in the Food Guide Pyramid. In practical terms, this works out in the following way. A young athlete consuming 2,500 calories a day needs on average about 1,250 carbohydrate calories daily, equivalent to about 312 grams (11 ounces) of carbohydrate food, or 6 to 11 servings.

For short, intense bursts of activity, such as sprints or weight-lifting events, athletes get their energy from glucose stored as glycogen in the muscles and liver. Longer events requiring sustained effort draw calories first from glycogen, then from body fat. Some athletes try the technique known as "carbohydrate loading" to boost their glycogen stores just before a major competition. The idea is to consume as many carbohydrates as possible while cutting down on the time spent training on the day before the event. Carbohydrate loading also requires drinking extra water and juices to prevent dehydration, because glycogen needs extra water for storage.

Although carbohydrate loading can help athletes taking part in endurance events lasting 90 minutes or longer, it is not recommended for shorter competitions or for athletes taking part in sports at the high-school level. Teenage athletes should follow the Food Guide Pyramid (see p. 90) to meet at least half of their daily energy requirements with carbohydrates.

A carbohydrate snack or a drink of juice right after a training session helps to replace the glycogen in muscles. Carbohydrates at the next meal will help to keep the muscles primed for training.

Protein

Protein is essential for growth, energy, and tissue repair. Athletic performance depends on muscle strength, and muscles are made of protein. But it's a mistake to think you can build up muscles by eating lots of protein. It's exercise, not dietary protein, that increases muscle mass.

The amount of protein adolescents need varies at different stages of development. As a rule, boys and girls between ages 11 and 14 need half a gram per pound of body weight daily. Thus, a young teenager weighing 110 pounds needs about 50 grams of protein a day. Between ages 15 and 18, the RDA drops slightly. As with all the essential nutrients, common sense is the rule: You don't have to weigh every gram on a scale. Each gram of protein provides 4 calories—the same as carbohydrates—and protein should make up about 10 to 12 percent of each day's calories.

The protein in foods of animal origin is termed complete or high-quality protein because it contains all the essential amino acids (see Chapter 6) in about the proportions humans need. Vegetable proteins are called incomplete because, except for soybeans, they have low levels of one or more essential amino acids. You don't have to eat animal products to obtain high-quality protein, however. People on vegetarian diets (see Chapter 14) take care of their protein needs by pairing plant foods that balance each other's shortfalls. Pairing foods in this way is called protein complementation. Eating a grain and a legume does the trick; beans and tortillas, a peanut butter sandwich on wheat bread, and black-eyed peas and rice are good examples of protein complementation. You can also compen-

PROTEIN AND CALORIE CONTENT OF FOODS MOST TEENAGERS LIKE TO EAT

Food	Protein content (grams)	Calorie average
Bagel (1 medium)	7	200
Bread, whole wheat, 1 slice	3	60–65
Cheese, processed, American (1 ounce)	6	105
Cheeseburger (4-ounce meat patty)	30	525
Lean meat, fish, or poultry (3-ounce serving)	22	180/120/140
Milk, skim—1% to 2%—whole (8 ounces)	8	85/100–120/150
Peanut butter (1 tablespoon)	5	95
Pizza, cheese (1 slice)	15	290
Taco	9	195
Yogurt, low-fat, coffee or vanilla (8 ounces)	8	195

sate for any lack in a plant-based food by adding a small amount of animal protein, such as in pasta with cheese or cereal with milk.

Water

Without water, the most abundant substance in the body, many of the biochemical processes that produce energy couldn't take place. Every cell is bathed in water, which carries nutrients around the body. Water helps regulate the body temperature. Finally, water flushes out the waste products left over from energy metabolism.

Water is lost through sweating, urination, and evaporation from the respiratory tract as a person breathes. During exercise, the rate of loss is faster as the athlete breathes faster and sweats more. Even more water is lost if exercise takes place in hot weather or in a warm indoor area. An athlete who loses too much water loses the ability to reg-ulate his body temperature and runs a risk of heat exhaustion and circulatory collapse. Adolescents competing in sports where weight is a factor, such as gymnastics and wrestling, may be pressured by coaches to "make weight" for an event. Wrestlers are particularly vulnerable because coaches demand that they train at one weight level and compete at another, lower one. Common practices to get the athlete to meet the required weight include restrictive dieting (for example, eating only bananas or oranges for several days in a row), water deprivation, and heavy workouts while wearing heat-retaining clothing. Such practices are dangerous—they have led to several deaths among college-level wrestlers.

Children with a history of eating disorders or chronic disease, such as diabetes or cystic fibrosis, should be especially careful about fluid loss. These teenagers sometimes fail to recognize sig-

Water is fine if children exercise for less than 3 hours in normal weather conditions. However, if an event lasts longer than 3 hours or the weather is hot and humid, an athlete may need to replace not only water but also the electrolytes—sodium, potassium, and chloride—that help regulate the body's balance of fluids. Athletes taking part in prolonged events should drink cool water or juice mixed with water. Commercial sports drinks are not necessary. Never use salt pills; they can be dangerous.

nals from the brain's thirst center, which may not function properly, and they can rapidly become dehydrated before they feel thirsty.

Thirst is not a reliable guide to the need for water. In fact, by the time a child feels thirsty he already may be seriously dehydrated. Young athletes taking part in games or practice should take regular breaks for water whether or not they feel thirsty. An adolescent approaching adult size should drink six to eight 8-ounce glasses of fluid a day—more during exercise and in hot weather—and consume plenty of fruits and vegetables, which have a high water content.

About 30 minutes before a practice or game, an athlete should drink 10 to 12 ounces of water or juice mixed with water, even if he doesn't feel thirsty. It doesn't matter if he feels temporarily "overhydrated." What the body can't use will soon pass out as urine. During games and practice, young athletes should take a break every 20 minutes to drink 3 or 4 ounces of water.

PMS and Sweets

Some adolescent girls have an irresistible craving for sweet foods and candy a few days before each menstrual period. Similar carbohydrate cravings occur in people who gain weight when under stress or while trying to give up smoking. Researchers found that women with severe premenstrual symptoms felt happier and calmer if their evening meals were high in carbohydrates and low in protein in the days preceding their periods. The women were less depressed, tense, and confused, and felt calmer and more alert than women who kept to their regular diet.

The researchers traced the explanation to serotonin, a brain chemical known to be involved in mood and appetite. Serotonin release is controlled by food intake; carbohydrates boost serotonin release whereas protein has no effect. Nicotine, like carbohydrates, increases brain serotonin while nicotine withdrawal has the opposite effect.

If your teenager is unusually tense or tearful around the time of her periods, she may feel better if her meals and snacks include more complex carbohydrates, such as pasta and grains. She should make a corresponding cut in her intake of animal protein and should avoid simple sugars,

▷ HIDDEN CAFFEINE

Your anxious, wakeful teenager may not be aware of how much caffeine she's consuming in the course of a day. Obvious sources include colas, coffee, and tea, including decaffeinated beverages. But there are also hidden ones, such as over-the-counter headache remedies and other kinds of soda pop.

A teenager who is used to a steady intake of caffeine may develop a caffeine-withdrawal headache a day or two after cutting back. Some complain of a weekend headache, which appears when a person who starts every weekday with a caffeine drink sleeps late on Saturday and misses the "dose" at the regular time. Once the caffeine habit is broken, caffeine-withdrawal headache should disappear within a week or two.

such as in candy and desserts, which often include hefty amounts of fat as well. In this way, she'll lift her mood and maintain balanced nutrition while avoiding extra, empty calories.

Teenage Jitters and Caffeine

Hearing sobs from her daughter's room, Robin Schneider knocked, then pushed open the door to find 17-year-old Jessica curled up in a fetal position on her bed.

"Something's really wrong with me, Mom," Jessica wailed. "My heart keeps racing out of control and sometimes I can't get my breath!"

To Robin—a trained nurse—the teenager looked distressed but not ill. Her temperature and color were normal and she had no chest pain. When Jessica mentioned that she had had several episodes of bringing up a sour, burning fluid and added that she couldn't get to sleep, Robin put two and two together.

Jessica had been meeting friends three or four times a week for iced caffè latte at the new coffee bar in town. She often drank a cola for an afternoon pick-me-up, despite her mother's suggestion that she drink juice instead. When she felt drowsy during morning classes, she drank a jolt of the new extra-caffeine soda that she and her classmates saw advertised on television. Also, to ease menstrual cramps, her mother had given the teenager several tablets of an over-the-counter headache remedy when she'd run out of her usual pain reliever.

Robin thought Jessica's problems might be caused by too much caffeine. Caffeine is a strong stimulant that can cause the heart to race, provoke stomach upsets, and—as Jessica was aware—prevent drowsiness. The effects may bring on a feeling of anxiety that makes it hard to breathe. Jessica was a slender girl, 5 feet 4 inches and 112 pounds. A rough tally of her recent intake showed that she was consuming enough caffeine each day to give a burly man the jitters.

▷ **WHAT MAKES A DIET VEGETARIAN?**

Vegetarians differ in degree, just as they differ in their reasons for adopting a vegetarian lifestyle. Partial or semivegetarians avoid some but not all animal products. They may eat chicken or fish and dairy products, but no red meat. Some eat fish but no poultry. Lacto-ovo-vegetarians eat eggs and dairy products but avoid all flesh; lacto-vegetarians don't eat eggs. Vegans follow a strict diet that excludes all foods derived from animals, including eggs and dairy products. Fruitarians eat only fruit, nuts and seeds, honey, whole grains, and olive oil. (For more details, see Chapter 14.)

Some people develop acne after consuming foods with a high iodine content. The amount of iodine required to trigger acne is many times the normal dietary level. There isn't enough iodine in seafood and iodized salt to cause skin problems, but acne has been linked to the high iodine levels in kelp, a seaweed extract sometimes included in sports drinks.

A few medications can also cause acne. Adolescents under treatment with certain steroids, antiepilepsy medications, or lithium should talk to their pediatricians about the effects of such medications on the skin.

Jessica promised to cut down on her iced caffe latte and order only the decaf version. She also agreed to drink juices and bottled waters instead of sodas. Finally, she planned to try getting up a quarter-hour earlier. That way she'd have time for breakfast.

Caffeine, a stimulant that works on the central nervous system, can stop a drowsy feeling and keep you alert. Too much, however, can cause palpitations (the feeling that your heart is racing or thumping hard), heartburn, sleeplessness, and a jittery, anxious feeling. The effect varies according to the size of the dose as well as the size of the consumer. Some people are more sensitive to caffeine while others build up a tolerance through regular use. A jittery, anxious teenager should cut back on colas and other sodas, coffee, and tea, including iced beverages, for a week or so. Even decaffeinated coffee and tea can deliver a substantial dose of caffeine. When a pain reliever is necessary, check the label to make sure it doesn't contain caffeine. If your teenager is still bothered by symptoms, talk to your pediatrician.

Fads and Diets

Teenage opinions about food may be based on concern for the environment and our role in it, on a humanitarian view of animal exploitation, or on the relationship between diet and health. In many cases, such opinions are well thought out and deserve respect. At times, adolescents may be pardoned for focusing on food as a symbol of everything that's wrong in their families if the table is usually laden with fat and lacking in fiber.

Parents can safely ignore faddish notions about food as long as the teenager continues to eat a balanced diet. Vegetarian diets, which are appealing to many, are so widely accepted that few consider them faddish any more (also see Chapter 14). Among adolescents, the most common reason for rejecting meat is an aversion to the exploitation of animals. Long-term vegetarians who maintain a proper nutritional balance have lower rates of several diseases that are associated with the typical Western high-fat, low-fiber diet. They are less likely to have high blood pressure and high cholesterol levels, and their weight is usually closer to a healthy ideal than that of meat eaters.

The more restricted the diet, the greater the risk of nutritional deficiency. Partial vegetarians usually have no difficulty getting a good balance of nutrients. They should take care, however, that complex carbohydrates make up the bulk of their diet. Some rely too much on dairy products and end up with a diet that's too high in fats and calories. All vegetarians should learn how to combine two or more carbohydrates to ensure an adequate

For a teenager being treated for acne, vitamin supplements could be not only unnecessary but dangerous as well. Certain acne treatments available by prescription are derived from vitamin A. This fat-soluble vitamin is stored in the body and can build up to toxic levels if too much is consumed.

A teenager who is eating a balanced diet based on the Food Guide Pyramid shouldn't need vitamin supplements. Taking a vitamin A supplement at the same time as an oral acne treatment could result in toxic levels, causing headaches, further skin and hair problems, and—in severe cases—liver and nerve damage.

intake of essential amino acids, the building blocks of protein.

Those who keep to a strict vegan diet must find alternative sources of vitamin D, important for healthy bones, and vitamin B_{12}, which is needed in all cells but especially for healthy blood. Humans can obtain some vitamin D from sunlight, but cannot absorb the B_{12} that occurs in small amounts in a few plant foods. Vegans of all ages should consume soy milk or cereals fortified with B_{12}. Without dairy foods, a vegan diet may also lack calcium. Your pediatrician or a qualified dietitian may recommend supplements to ensure that your child has adequate intakes of vitamins, calcium, iron, and zinc.

Any adolescent planning to embark on a diet should first talk with a pediatrician, who may recommend books on nutrition or provide a referral to a nutrition counselor.

Image and Eating Disorders

Teenagers sometimes develop notions about food that are based on a distorted body image and an overconcern with reshaping it. Food fads and refusals are not unusual during adolescence and usually pass quickly. Eating disorders, however, are serious problems that are associated with health risks and emotional disturbances. These disorders usually affect girls, but are also seen in boys. They are not always easy to detect, because adolescents with eating disorders may maintain normal weight or wear bulky clothing to disguise weight loss. The major types of eating disorder involve self-starvation, gorging, binge-eating, and purging. (Also see Chapter 10.)

A teenager with an eating disorder urgently needs professional help. If your child has had an unusual weight loss or gain, seems obsessed with food preparation or dieting, or is exercising compulsively for hours on end, talk to your pediatrician.

Food and Adolescent Acne

More than 80 percent of teenagers have acne, so if your young person manages to get through adolescence with no more than a couple of skin blem-

People under stress often crave chocolate and sweets. After eating candy, they have an acne outbreak, then mistakenly associate the candies with the acne outbreak but overlook the real culprit, stress.

"Life without Brussels sprouts is still worth living, but life without chocolate—that's another story!"

ishes, he's one of the lucky few. Contrary to what most people believe, acne is not caused by chocolate, fried foods, candies, or anything else in a normal diet. It's not the result of constipation, nor is it a sign of sexual activity or the lack of it. Instead, it's due to increased levels of certain hormones, which stimulate the sebaceous glands to step up production of sebum, an oily secretion that lubricates and protects the skin. Sebum, together with cast-off skin cells and other debris, blocks skin follicles, which can become infected or inflamed. The increase in sebum production may occur as early as 2 years before any other signs of puberty, and boys and girls as young as age 9 may have skin bumps and coarsened pores, especially in areas where sebaceous glands are numerous, such as around the nose and the middle of the face.

There's often a tendency for acne to run in families. Most cases are mild, and pimples and zits don't usually leave permanent scars if the lesions are left alone. Over-the-counter lotions containing benzoyl peroxide can be helpful for minor blemishes. Your pediatrician or dermatologist can prescribe treatment for more severe or persistent acne.

Although there's no proven link between diet and acne, it won't hurt to avoid chocolate and sugary or fatty foods if your teenager believes they trigger blemishes. Indeed, it may be better for her health. Adolescence is an inherently stressful time, and if stress triggers your child's acne,

measures to help her control stress may also help cut down on acne outbreaks.

Oily creams and lotions can block skin follicles and promote sebum buildup. Teenagers should avoid oil-based skin and hair cosmetics and use nonperfumed, water-based products.

Alcohol and Adolescents

Many young people start using alcohol during the early adolescent years, and girls, on the whole, seem to experiment with alcohol and drugs at an earlier age than boys. If alcohol were not in the picture, many tragedies among young Americans could be prevented, including car crashes, drownings, fatal falls, homicides, and suicides. Alcohol loosens inhibitions and increases the risk of irresponsible sexual behavior that can result in unplanned pregnancies and sexually transmitted diseases.

 SMOKING AND TEENAGERS

Adolescents continue to smoke despite overwhelming evidence that cigarettes are harmful. Girls, in particular, take up smoking as a method of weight control. What they don't know is that cigarette smoking partly suppresses the female hormone estrogen, which influences fat deposits in women. Women who smoke, therefore, tend to acquire fat on the abdomen—in the male pattern—instead of on the thighs and hips. So, although a girl smokes to keep her weight down, she's redistributing her body fat in a way that can give her a pot belly.

Many adolescents don't continue to drink after an initial experimentation. For those who persist, however, the risks are great. Adolescents on the whole are smaller and lighter—and thus get drunk faster—than adults. Some adolescents are at higher risk than others for becoming alcoholics. Genetic and psychological factors such as depression can make a susceptible teenager dependent on alcohol, and dependency can develop in much less time than with an adult.

Parents may feel torn by two apparent choices. Should they gradually introduce their under-age children to alcohol by allowing beer and wine on special occasions in a controlled family environment? Or should they forbid any exposure to alcohol until the legal drinking age?

The American Academy of Pediatrics warns that children and adolescents should not be allowed to use alcohol or nicotine, or any drugs except for prescribed medications. The Academy urges parents who drink to do so safely and in moderation, and to keep alcohol out of children's reach. It discourages the practice of giving alcohol to children, although it acknowledges that some parents may accept the supervised use of wine in religious ceremonies. The Academy supports a policy of "zero tolerance" against alcohol, tobacco, and all drugs in schools and at school-related events. This ban should extend equally to students and staff. Driver's licenses should be automatically suspended—or not granted—for minors convicted of violating alcohol and drug laws.

Young people may be introduced to controlled drinking in the family home after they have reached the legal age.

FOOD PROBLEMS THAT TEENAGERS' PARENTS WORRY ABOUT

My son wants to try carbohydrate loading for his high-school field day. He's been picked for the four-man relay and may also compete in the long jump. Is carbo loading all he cracks it up to be?
While carbohydrate loading can help mature athletes taking part in endurance events lasting 90 minutes or longer, it is not recommended for shorter events or for teenagers taking part in sports at the high-school level. (Read about how to feed your teenage athlete on p. 79.)

My daughter often complains of a persistent, dull headache after she sleeps late on weekends. Is it because she sleeps too much?
Your daughter may be getting a caffeine-withdrawal headache. It happens when a person who is used to starting the day with a caffeinated drink sleeps late and misses the regular "dose." If she cuts down on caffeine (cola and coffee, for example) for a week or two and doesn't oversleep, she may break her caffeine dependence and get rid of the headache.

(For more about hidden caffeine and the symptoms it causes, turn to p. 83.)

My daughter has acne. Is it because she's overweight and keeps sneaking chocolate bars and French fries?
What your daughter eats has no effect on acne, but stress and hormones do. She should talk to her pediatrician about weight control, and ask for a referral to a dermatologist to treat her skin problems. (Read more about food and adolescent acne on p. 85.)

I'm afraid my teenager is heading for osteoporosis because she won't drink milk. She says it's got too many calories. How can I get her to eat more calcium?
Serve low-fat and nonfat milk, yogurt, and other dairy products. These have just as much calcium as the whole-milk versions. There are also ways to get calcium other than from dairy products. (Read about dietary calcium and healthy bones on p. 76.)

We keep reading about teenagers being injured while DWI. Couldn't a lot of these tragedies be prevented if parents taught youngsters to drink responsibly at home?
Only one factor has been found to reduce alcohol-related accidents among teenagers and that's abstinence. The accident rate went down after the legal drinking age was raised in all states. Don't allow your youngsters to drink alcohol before they reach the legal age, and teach them never, ever to drink and drive (see p. 87).

My son looks pale and washed out. Could it be because he won't eat red meat?
A properly balanced vegetarian diet can provide plenty of iron without the saturated fat in red meat. (Read about increasing iron absorption on p. 74 and vegetarian diets in Chapter 14.) If you suspect your son is anemic, arrange an appoinment with your pediatrician.

CHAPTER 6

Nutrition Basics

There's nothing magic about the Food Guide Pyramid (see p. 90), and it doesn't require special memorization or complicated math. All you have to remember is that the breads, cereals, grains, and pasta at the base should form the bulk of your child's diet, providing the greatest number of daily servings. Vegetables and fruits follow closely on the next level. We need fewer servings of the dairy foods and meat-fish-egg-legume (protein) group one level up. Finally, the added fats and sugars (simple carbohydrates) on top are optional and should be eaten sparingly, like mayonnaise on a sandwich or jelly on toast.

It's not necessary to eat the exact number of servings from each group every day. Rather, intake should average out to the portions indicated over a period of 1 to 2 weeks. The Pyramid builders recommend that everyone consume a range of portions from each of the five groups to ensure a healthy intake of calories along with all the essential nutrients, including carbohydrates, fiber, protein, fats, vitamins, and minerals. Although your child may have a strong dislike for one or several foods within a particular group, it's important to find foods he will eat in order to obtain the nutrients the group provides. If your child absolutely refuses all foods in a group (this is so rare it almost never happens), ask your pediatrician to refer you to a dietitian who can advise on substitutes to make up for any nutritional shortfall.

At first, the Pyramid recommendations may look like far more than anyone could possibly eat, with 5 of this and 11 of that. However, one area where the Pyramid asks us to adjust our thinking is in picturing portions instead of platefuls. Even for adults, the individual portions are modest. For example, a portion is $1/2$ cup of cooked pasta or rice, not a bowlful; or 2 to 3 ounces of lean meat (about the size of a deck of cards). Obviously, a person with a moderate appetite can eat much more than $1/2$ cup of cooked pasta at a meal, and a single plateful may include several portions of one or several foods. Children's portions should be scaled according to the three A's: Age, Appetite, and Activity level (see table, p. 92).

Notice that the portion size for young children is smaller than for older ones. It's best to start small and offer modest portions that children can easily manage, with second helpings if they ask for them. Large portions can be overwhelming and

Lots from the bottom, less from the middle, and a little from the top: That's the lesson of the Food Guide Pyramid for healthy food choices. Schools use the Pyramid to teach children the principles of healthy nutrition starting as early as kindergarten. Many food manufacturers include the Pyramid on package labels to show how their products fit into the overall scheme of nutrition. When shopping with your children, use these labels to help them see where their supermarket selections fit, or don't fit, in a healthy eating plan. It's also a good idea to post a Pyramid on your refrigerator door as a handy guide for meal planning.

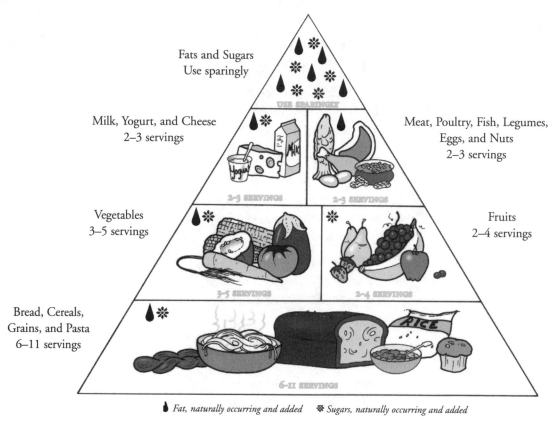

Fats and Sugars
Use sparingly

Milk, Yogurt, and Cheese
2–3 servings

Meat, Poultry, Fish, Legumes,
Eggs, and Nuts
2–3 servings

Vegetables
3–5 servings

Fruits
2–4 servings

Bread, Cereals,
Grains, and Pasta
6–11 servings

USE SPARINGLY

2–3 SERVINGS *2–3 SERVINGS*

3–5 SERVINGS *2–4 SERVINGS*

6–11 SERVINGS

🌢 *Fat, naturally occurring and added* ❋ *Sugars, naturally occurring and added*

RECOMMENDED SERVING SIZES: *Bread: 1 slice* • *Cereal, pasta, rice: 1 ounce* • *Vegetables: ½ cup*
Fruit: 1 medium piece, e.g., 1 apple • *Milk, yogurt: 1 cup* • *Cheese: 1½ ounces* • *Meat, poultry, fish: 2–3 ounces*

The Food Guide Pyramid is an outline to follow so that a week's food intake averages out on a daily basis to the servings shown. The number of servings for each food group is calculated for a theoretical average American.

take away a child's appetite. It's also important to remember that the Pyramid is a guide, not a prescription. Children may not eat all the servings from each group every day. However, as the Pyramid suggests, most of their food should come from the carbohydrates at the base.

Start with Carbohydrates

Foods from grains, such as breads, pasta, cereal, and brown rice, are packed with starches (complex carbohydrates), the best source of energy for active, growing bodies. Carbohydrates should make up 50 to 60 percent of the diet by age 5.

Foods in this group provide starch, protein, iron (a good source, though less fully absorbed than the iron in animal foods), most of the B vitamins—which are needed for the proper functioning of many enzymes that convert food to energy, as well as for a healthy nervous system—and vitamin K, needed for normal blood clotting and bone metabolism.

In the liver, carbohydrates are converted to

glucose, an important energy source for most tissues, especially the brain and nervous system. Glucose is stored in the liver and muscles in the form of glycogen. Our bodies also contain carbohydrates in many different forms, including hormones, enzymes, and supporting structures in the connective tissues.

As we understand more about how our bodies work and the importance of avoiding unnecessary fats to prevent heart disease, cancer, and other ills, we have shed the outdated view that starches are heavy and fattening. Grain dishes are low in fat unless large amounts of fats and oils are used in preparation. Pasta, rice, and other grain-based staples can be mixed with vegetables and moderate portions from the protein and dairy groups to provide a balanced meal. When consumed together with other plant foods (a grain plus a legume, such as whole-wheat bread with peanut butter, or rice and beans), grains are a good source of protein. In addition, eating a grain together with a modest serving of an animal food (such as in pizza, or rice topped with chili con carne) enhances our ability to absorb iron from the plant food. Consuming citrus or another food rich in vitamin C at the same meal also increases the absorption of plant iron. Whole grains (whole-wheat bread, brown rice) include fiber as a bonus.

Fiber

Dietary fiber is made up of carbohydrate compounds that cannot be digested, such as cellulose and pectin. Fiber is present in the cell walls of all plants, but is not found in any foods obtained from animals. Insoluble fiber, such as in wheat bran, fruit skins, and corn kernels, passes through the intestine unchanged. Soluble fiber, found in oat bran or the pectin that helps jam to jell, expands and becomes gel-like on contact with water.

Although we cannot absorb fiber, it is an essential part of a healthy diet. People who eat a lot of fiber are less likely to be obese, have heart disease, or develop problems affecting the bowel, including constipation and cancer. Fiber makes the stools larger, softer, and easier to pass. Studies show that people who consume a diet rich in soluble fiber have lower blood cholesterol levels.

Phytate compounds in fiber may reduce the absorption of some minerals, especially zinc, which is essential for sexual maturation, and calcium, which is needed by almost every organ system, but especially the bones and teeth. However, phytate in whole wheat is destroyed by

 COLOR ME NUTRITIOUS

Encourage your child to make colorful platefuls, with vegetables and fruits in a range of reds, yellows, and greens. The more color on the plate, the more varied and comprehensive the selection of nutrients is likely to be.

yeast fermentation, and most bread consumed in the United States is made with yeast. Thus, eating yeast-risen bread blocks any harmful effect from phytate and lets the body absorb calcium. In addition, a high-fiber diet is unlikely to lead to mineral deficiencies as long as children eat a variety of foods to provide many different sources of nutrients.

Your child's fiber intake from all sources—whole grains, vegetables, fruits—should equal his or her age plus 5; thus, for a 9-year old, 9 + 5 = 14 grams a day, up to a maximum of 35 grams a day. Recommendations that children should eat only low-calorie, high-fiber foods are not to be trusted.

	1 to 3 years one serving	4 to 6 years one serving	7 to 10 years one serving

Grains
6 to 11 servings/
day
	Bread, $1/2$ slice
	Cereal, rice, pasta,
	  cooked, $1/4$ cup
	Cereal, dry, $1/3$ cup
	Crackers, 2 to 3
		Bread, $1/2$ slice
		Cereal, rice, pasta,
		  cooked, $1/3$ cup
		Cereal, dry, $1/2$ cup
		Crackers, 3 to 4
			Bread, 1 slice
			Cereal, rice, pasta,
			  cooked, $1/2$ cup
			Cereal, dry, $3/4$ to 1 cup
			Crackers, 4 to 5

Vegetables
2–3 servings/day
	Vegetables, cooked,
	  $1/4$ cup
		Vegetables, cooked,
		  $1/4$ cup
		Salad, $1/2$ cup
			Vegetables, cooked,
			  $1/2$ cup
			Salad, 1 cup

Fruits
2–3 servings/day
	Fruit, cooked or canned,
	  $1/4$ cup;
	Fruit, fresh, $1/2$ piece
	Juice, $1/4$ cup
		Fruit, cooked or canned,
		  $1/4$ cup
		Fruit, fresh, $1/2$ piece
		Juice, $1/3$ cup
			Fruit, cooked or canned,
			  $1/3$ cup
			Fruit, fresh, 1 piece
			Juice, $1/2$ cup

Dairy 2–3 servings/day	Milk, $1/2$ cup Cheese, $1/2$ ounce Yogurt, $1/3$ cup	Milk, $1/2$ cup Cheese, 1 ounce Yogurt, $1/2$ cup	Milk, 1 cup Cheese, 1 ounce Yogurt, $3/4$ to 1 cup

Meats and other
proteins
2 servings/day
	Meat, fish, poultry, tofu,
	  1 ounce (2 1-inch cubes)
	Beans, dried, cooked,
	  $1/4$ cup
	Egg, $1/2$
		Meat, fish, poultry, tofu,
		  1 ounce (2 1-inch cubes)
		Beans, dried, cooked,
		  $1/3$ cup
		Egg, 1
			Meat, fish, poultry, tofu,
			  2 to 3 ounces
			Beans, dried, cooked,
			  $1/2$ cup
			Eggs, 1 or 2

Children need calories for growth and activity, and while fiber is good, too much of it could prevent a child from absorbing essential nutrients.

Vegetables

Parents worry more about their children's poor consumption of vegetables than any other food group, and with good reason. Surveys show that many, if not most, school-age children do not eat two to three daily servings of vegetables, even though the recommended amounts add up to only $1/2$ to $3/4$ cup for ages 4 to 6, and $1 1/2$ cups for 7- to 10-year-olds.

Vegetables are the most important source of beta carotene (which our bodies convert to vitamin A for healthy skin, glands, immune system, and eye function) and many other vitamins and phytochemicals—naturally occurring plant compounds that are believed to fight cancer and other diseases. Vegetables also provide plenty of fiber.

Vegetables and fruits are excellent sources of folic acid, also called folate or folacin, a vitamin that is needed to make the genetic material (DNA and RNA) in our cells, as well as for the production of red blood cells (also see pp. 97-99). A good supply of folic acid is essential at every age. If women have low levels of folic acid at the time of conception, their babies run an increased risk of serious birth defects involving the nervous system and spine, as well as many other organs. Folic acid is particularly important, therefore, for teenage girls, to ensure that they will be properly prepared when the time comes to plan their families. A child who consumes five fruits and vegetables a day usually gets enough folic acid. Other good sources are organ meats, eggs, chickpeas (garbanzo beans), nuts, and breads, crackers, and pasta made with whole wheat.

The National Cancer Institute urges everyone, adult or child, to consume at least two or three servings of vegetables a day, adding up to the magic five a day of vegetables and fruits recommended to keep healthy and resist illness. The five should include at least one choice rich in vitamin A, at least one rich in vitamin C, at least one high-fiber selection, and something from the cabbage family (these vegetables are called cruciferous because their flower petals grow in cross form) several times a week.

With a bit of creativity, it's not difficult to get even a vegetable-hater to eat at least the minimum number of daily servings. A child who doesn't enjoy cooked vegetables may happily snack on carrot sticks or a selection of vegetables served with a low-fat dip. Pasta can be dressed with a fresh vegetable sauce; pizza is colorful, appetizing, and healthful when topped with vegetables such as green peppers, mushrooms, asparagus, or broccoli rabe, in addition to tomato sauce.

Fruits

Whole fruits and fruit juices provide many essential vitamins and minerals, together with a variety of disease-fighting phytochemicals like those in vegetables, and fiber. Above all, fruits are our most important source of vitamin C. We need this vitamin to produce collagen, the connective substance that holds cells together and helps maintain blood vessels, bones and cartilage, and teeth.

Protein and Amino Acids

We eat protein foods to obtain 20 amino acids, building blocks that we remake into our bodies' own unique proteins and other compounds, including the neurotransmitters that carry communications between cells. Nine of the amino acids (see table p. 95) are called essential, because we cannot manufacture them ourselves and must obtain them from the foods we eat. The remaining 11 are called nonessential because our bodies can make them, even if they are lacking from the diet.

Body proteins and other compounds are con-

WHEN IS VITAMIN C NOT QUITE VITAMIN C?

Fruits provide a good example of the importance of obtaining nutrients from foods and not from supplements. For proper nutrition, we need nutrients such as vitamins and minerals in two forms—oxidized and reduced—and in balance with other substances in the same food. Supplements contain only an extract of an isolated nutrient, without the other naturally occurring substances that either promote its effects or keep them in check.

For example, to get the maximum benefit from vitamin C, we need to consume it in two forms: ascorbic acid, the reduced form, and dehydroascorbic acid, the oxidized form. Fruits and vegetables provide a balance of the two forms of the vitamin; supplements contain only ascorbic acid.

stantly broken down and rebuilt in a process called protein turnover. The turnover rate is highest in children, who are still growing and maturing. We need a steady supply of amino acids to make and repair protein, because our bodies cannot store excess amino acids from food. Therefore, the daily protein intake should be spaced over several meals throughout the day. This is especially important for children. However, while protein remains an essential nutrient throughout life, the need for protein decreases with age. For example, the amount of protein required for growth drops from about 56 percent of the amount consumed daily by a newborn to about 5 percent of daily consumption by age 5. At any age, the ideal protein is one that contains all the amino acids in the required amounts, without any excess. For babies up to age 1, breastmilk contains the ideal amino acid balance. Slightly different patterns are recommended for the changing growth rates from 1 to 6 years, and again from 6 to 13 years. After age

TOO MUCH OF A GOOD THING

The high amount of protein in the average American diet shows that we consume far more than we need. The effects of too much protein over a long period are not known, but may contribute to hardening of the arteries and kidney disease. Too much protein in the diet may also lead to excessive loss of calcium in the urine, which increases the risk of osteoporosis, or weakening of the bones, in later life. An extremely high protein intake can increase fluid loss, especially during activity in warm conditions, and lead to dehydration. Young athletes should eat a normal diet with moderate amounts of protein, avoid protein supplements, and drink plenty of water (see also p. 80), especially when they exercise in warm weather.

13, the requirements are the same as for adults.

Animal foods, such as milk, meat, and fish, provide all the essential amino acids in the right proportions for humans. Therefore, proteins from such sources are called complete. Grains and legumes—plants whose seeds grow in pods, such as peas, beans, and peanuts—are also good sources of protein. Plant proteins are called incomplete, because they have low levels of one or more essential amino acids. The only known exception is soy protein, which has a pattern of amino acids closer to animal proteins than other plant proteins.

This doesn't mean that people have to eat animal protein to be healthy. Well-informed vegetarians (also see Chapter 14) know that it's a fairly simple matter to match up plant foods that provide complementary proteins; in other words, one food makes up for the amino acid that the other lacks. For example, cereal grains such as wheat have low levels of the amino acid lysine but plenty of methionine. By contrast, legumes such as beans, peas, and peanuts have good levels of lysine but little methionine. Thus, a combination as simple as whole-wheat bread with peanut butter provides a complete protein, because the methionine in the wheat complements the lysine in the peanuts. In addition, eating even a small amount of animal protein, such as meat or cheese, with a plant-based food will make up for any essential amino acid lacking in the plant food. This is the system that much healthy ethnic cooking is based on; think of black beans and rice, hopping john, tortillas with beans, lentil soup with sausage, and pasta e fagioli.

The advantage of proteins obtained from grains and vegetables is that most are naturally low in fat, in contrast to proteins in animal foods, which are "packaged" with substantial

ESSENTIAL AMINO ACIDS	NONESSENTIAL AMINO ACIDS
Isoleucine	Glycine
Leucine	Glutamic acid
Lysine	Arginine*
Methionine	Aspartic acid
Phenylalanine	Proline
Threonine	Alanine
Tryptophan	Serine
Valine	Tyrosine**
Histidine	Cysteine**
	Asparagine
	Glutamine

*May become essential if the body cannot manufacture it because of illness or prematurity.

**Essential for premature infants and healthy newborns, who cannot synthesize it.

amounts of fat, including saturated fat. Peanuts are an exception—they contain a high proportion of fat, including saturated fat. (When opening a new jar of "natural" peanut butter, pour off the oil at the top.)

As far as protein is concerned, an ounce of meat, poultry, or fish is equivalent to 1 egg, $1/2$ cup cooked beans, or 2 tablespoons peanut butter. The fat and cholesterol content varies, of course, according to the source.

Milk and Milk-Based Foods

Milk is children's best source of calcium, and is an important source of protein, riboflavin (vitamin

To create a substitute for butter, vegetable oils are put through a process called hydrogenation that makes them firm and resistant to spoilage (also see Chapter 13). However, hydrogenated or "trans" fats not only spread like butter, but also share some of the undesirable properties of saturated fats. They appear to interfere with the removal of cholesterol from the blood, and may contribute to heart disease and certain cancers. To lower your children's consumption of saturated fats, avoid trans fats and use liquid oils and soft tub margarines instead. Always check labels for trans fat content.

B_2), and many other nutrients. Vitamin D is added to milk to prevent rickets, and vitamin A is added to skim milk to replace what's lost when fat is skimmed off. Butter and cheese provide all the nutrients of milk and yogurt in a more concentrated form. Portions should be modest, because the fat content is high. For children younger than 2 years, fats should make up about half of the total calorie intake. For that reason they should drink whole milk and eat whole-milk yogurt and cheeses. After age 2, children may drink low-fat or nonfat milk and eat low-fat or nonfat yogurt.

Adolescent girls tend to shun milk because they think it contains too many calories. They drink fruit juice and soft drinks instead. As a result, many of them have diets that are seriously lacking in calcium and may lead to osteoporosis once they enter the middle years. Girls should keep up their calcium intake by consuming non-fat milk and low-fat yogurt, which provide the same nutrients as whole milk without unnecessary fat. Remind your daughters and their friends that nonfat milk contains fewer calories than many juices and soft drinks.

Fats and Fatty Acids

Fats are the most misunderstood of all the food groups. They are essential to good health and they add greatly to the pleasure of eating. They impart a pleasing texture and consistency to foods and, because they slow down the stomach's rate of emptying, add to our feeling of fullness and satisfaction. In our bodies, fats are vital components of the cell membranes. They enable us to absorb the fat-soluble vitamins A, D, E, and K, and play a role in normal blood clotting. Fat is necessary for production of the various hormones that help boys and girls mature and that keep adult bodies functioning properly. Above all, fat is the body's most economical method of storing energy.

Fats should constitute half of the daily intake of calories by children younger than 2. After age 2, fat consumption should be reduced until it settles at no more than 30 percent of total daily calories.

For reasons that have not yet been fully explained, highly saturated fat interferes with the removal of cholesterol from the blood and thus contributes to increases in blood cholesterol levels. Over a long period, high blood cholesterol can increase the risk of developing atherosclerosis—a buildup of fatty deposits on the insides of the arteries—and heart attacks. Researchers have found the fatty streaks that come before the fat deposits in the arteries of 7 percent of children starting at age 10, and in more than twice as many children after age 15. They advise cutting saturated fat to one third of the total fat intake;

that is, a maximum of 10 percent of the calories consumed in a day.

The terms saturated, unsaturated, polyunsaturated, and monounsaturated merely refer to the number and arrangement of hydrogen atoms in each molecule of fat. In general, saturated fats are those that stay firm at room temperature. Animal fats, such as butter and lard, are good examples. Some vegetable oils, including coconut and palm oils, also contain a high proportion of saturated fats. Monounsaturated fats, such as olive oil, are liquid at room temperature, but become firmer on cooling. Polyunsaturated fats remain liquid even when refrigerated.

About half the fat in red meat is saturated; poultry fat is less so. Two thirds of the fat in full-fat dairy foods is saturated. Fish fats for the most part are polyunsaturated. If they were not, the body fat would harden at the low temperatures of a fish's normal habitat and the fish couldn't swim.

Vitamin	Effect	Signs of deficiency	Signs of overdose	Good sources
Fat-soluble vitamins: Vitamin A	Keeps skin, hair, nails healthy. Helps maintain gums, glands, bones, teeth. Helps prevent infection. Promotes eye function; prevents night blindness.	Night blindness; dry eyes; growth delay in children; dry, rough skin; low resistance to infection.	Headaches; blurred vision; fatigue; diarrhea; dry, cracked skin, rash, itch; hair loss; bone and joint pain; liver damage; irregular periods; birth defects if taken during pregnancy.	Milk and dairy foods; fortified cereals; green and yellow vegetables; deep yellow or orange fruits; organ meats.
Vitamin D	Helps build and maintain bones; needed for calcium absorption.	Rickets in children; osteomalacia (bone softening) in adults; osteoporosis (thinning and weakening of bones).	Calcium deposits, mainly in heart, kidneys, blood vessels; weak bones; high blood pressure; high blood cholesterol levels; diarrhea; drowsiness; headache.	Egg yolks; fish oils; fortified milk and butter; exposure to sunlight without sunscreen.
Vitamin E	Helps form red blood cells, muscles, other tissues; antioxidant; stabilizes cell membranes; preserves fatty acids.	Blood problems in premature infants; neurological problems in older children and adults.	Bleeding; changes in white blood cell function.	Poultry, seafood; green leafy vegetables; wheat germ; whole grains, seeds, nuts; butter; liver; egg yolk.
Vitamin K	Needed for normal blood clotting; helps maintain healthy bones.	Excessive bleeding; liver damage.	Jaundice (yellowing) in infants; blood changes.	Produced by intestinal bacteria; cow's milk; green leafy vegetables; pork, liver; oats, wheat bran, whole grains.

Vitamin	Effect	Signs of deficiency	Signs of overdose	Good sources
Water-soluble vitamins:				
Thiamin (vitamin B_1)	Promotes carbohydrate metabolism; needed for normal appetite, digestion, nerve function; enhances energy.	Anxiety, depression; nausea; muscle cramps; appetite loss; in extreme cases, muscle-wasting disease.	Too much of one B vitamin may cause deficiency of others (excess B_1 can interfere with B_2 and B_6).	Pork, seafood; fortified grains, cereals.
Riboflavin (vitamin B_2)	Needed for all food metabolism; maintains mucous membranes; helps maintain vision; facilitates release of energy to cells.	Cracks and sores around mouth and nose; sensitivity to light; difficulty eating and swallowing.	Can interfere with B_1 and B_6.	Organ meats, beef, lamb, dark meat of poultry; dairy foods; fortified cereals, grains; dark green leafy vegetables.
Niacin/ nicotinic acid (vitamin B_3)	Needed in many enzymes that convert food to energy; promotes normal appetite and digestion; promotes nerve function.	Diarrhea, mouth sores. In extreme deficiency: pellagra, with skin rash, inflammation of mucous membranes, diarrhea, mental symptoms.	Ulcers; liver damage; hot flushes; high blood sugar and uric acid; disturbances of heart rhythm; itchy skin.	Produced by intestinal bacteria; poultry, seafood; seeds, nuts, peanuts, potatoes; fortified whole-grain breads and cereals.
Pantothenic acid (vitamin B_5)	Needed to break down food into molecular forms required by body; involved in the manufacture of adrenal hormones and chemicals that regulate nerve function.	Unknown in humans, except when induced experimentally.	May increase need for thiamin; megadoses may cause diarrhea and water retention.	Found in almost all plant and animal foods.
Pyridoxine (vitamin B_6)	Required for metabolism and absorption of protein; important in carbohydrate metabolism; helps form red blood cells; promotes nerve function.	Depression, mental confusion; inflammation of mucous membranes of mouth; itchy scaling patches on skin; convulsions in infants.	Can lead to destruction of sensory nerves, with loss of feeling in limbs, fingers, and toes.	Meats, fish, poultry; grains, cereals; spinach, sweet and white potatoes; bananas, prunes, watermelon.

Saturation doesn't change the number of calories. All fats—butter, margarine, salad oil—contain 9 calories per gram, or between 240 and 250 calories per ounce.

Vitamins

Vitamins are organic substances that are required for the body's metabolic processes. We need only minute amounts of vitamins, but if we don't get

Vitamin	Effect	Signs of deficiency	Signs of overdose	Good sources
Water-soluble vitamins (cont.): Vitamin B_{12} (cobalamin)	Helps build genetic material (nucleic acid) required by all cells; helps form red blood cells.	Anemia and nerve damage (deficiency is rare except in strict vegetarians who eat no foods of animal origin; the B_{12} that occurs in a few plant foods cannot be absorbed by humans).	Does not occur except in infants with a rare genetic disorder.	All foods of animal origin, including meats, poultry, eggs, seafood, dairy foods.
Biotin, a B vitamin	Required for glucose metabolism and formation of certain fatty acids; plays an essential part in many bodily processes.	Rare except in infants. Scaling skin; muscle pain; fatigue; loss of appetite; sleeplessness.	See vitamin B_1.	Produced by intestinal bacteria. Also obtained from meats, poultry, fish, eggs; nuts, seeds, legumes; vegetables.
Folic acid (folate, folacin), a B vitamin	Needed to make genetic material (DNA, RNA); needed for manufacture of red blood cells.	Anemia; gastrointestinal upsets, diarrhea, weight loss; bleeding gums; irritability; birth defects if levels are low in pregnancy.	Convulsions in epileptics (can interfere with anticonvulsant medication); megadoses can interfere with zinc absorption.	Poultry, liver; dark green leafy vegetables; legumes; fortified whole-grain breads, cereals; oranges, grapefruit.
Vitamin C (ascorbic acid)	Helps bind cells together; strengthens blood vessel walls; may have antihistaminic effect against common cold symptoms.	Bleeding gums, loose teeth; bruising; dry, rough skin; slow healing; appetite loss; scurvy in extreme cases.	Kidney stones; oxalate deposits in heart and other tissues; urinary tract irritation; diarrhea; anemia.	Citrus fruits; strawberries; cantaloupe, watermelon; sweet potatoes; cabbage, cauliflower, broccoli; plantains; snow peas.

Basalt Regional Library
99 Midland Avenue
Basalt CO 81621

enough, signs and symptoms of vitamin deficiency appear.

Thirteen vitamins are known to be essential for human health, although there may be others still unidentified. Daily requirements have been established for 11 of them. We obtain most of our vitamins from food (see the table beginning on p. 97 for the characteristics, effects, and sources of vitamins). However, vitamin D can be made in the skin with exposure to sunlight for 10 to 30 minutes a day, and the B vitamins biotin and nicotinic acid, as well as vitamin K, are made by bacteria normally present in the intestine.

Vitamins are grouped according to how they are absorbed by the body. Vitamins A, D, E, and K are absorbed in the presence of fat or bile and are stored in fat. Therefore, they are known as fat-soluble vitamins. The eight B vitamins and vitamin C are water soluble and do not require fat for

Mineral	Effect	Signs of deficiency	Signs of overdose	Good sources
Calcium	Builds bones, teeth; promotes nerve and muscle function; helps blood to clot; helps activate enzymes that convert food into energy.	Rickets (weak, deformed bones) in children; osteomalacia and osteoporosis (softening and thinning of bones) in adults.	Kidney stones and calcium deposits in tissues; mental confusion; muscle and abdominal pain; interferes with absorption of iron and other minerals.	Milk and dairy foods; canned fish (salmon, sardines) with bones; oysters; broccoli; tofu (bean curd).
Phosphorus	Works with calcium to build and maintain bones and teeth; needed by certain enzymes to convert food into energy; promotes nerve and muscle function; helps maintain body's chemical balance.	Weakness, bone pain (deficiency is rare).	Reduces blood calcium levels.	Dairy products; egg yolks; meat, poultry, fish; legumes.
Magnesium	Activates enzymes needed to release energy in body; promotes bone growth; needed to make cells and genetic material.	Muscle weakness, twitching, cramps; disturbances of heart rhythm (deficiencies rare in healthy children).	Imbalance between calcium and magnesium, leading to nervous system disorders.	Green leafy vegetables; beans; nuts; fortified whole-grain cereals and breads; shellfish.
Iron	Essential to make hemoglobin, the red oxygen-carrying pigment in blood, and myoglobin, a pigment that stores oxygen in muscles.	Anemia, with weakness, fatigue, shortness of breath.	Toxic buildup in liver, pancreas, heart; diabetes; liver disease; disturbances of heart rhythm; interference with zinc absorption.	Red meat, liver; fish, shellfish; legumes; fortified breads, cereals; dried apricots.

absorption. Our bodies store enough vitamins to meet general daily requirements, with a little extra in case the dietary supply should fail. The main storehouse is the liver, which absorbs and stores excess nutrients from the blood, and then releases into the blood those nutrients that are not supplied in adequate amounts by the diet.

Contrary to what advertisements claim, healthy children do not need vitamin supplements to make up for nutrients lacking in their food. Nor do they need a set dose of vitamins every day. As with other trace nutrients, what's important is that the average food consumption over a week or two includes a variety of foods to provide all the essential vitamins. It is always better to get vitamins from food than in pill

Mineral	Effect	Signs of deficiency	Signs of overdose	Good sources
Zinc	Needed in more than 100 enzymes instrumental in digestion and metabolism; essential for sexual maturation.	Slow wound healing; appetite loss; delayed growth and sexual development in children.	Nausea, vomiting, abdominal pain, gastric bleeding.	Beef, liver; oysters; yogurt; fortified cereals, wheat germ.
Selenium	Interacts with vitamin E to prevent breakdown of fats and body chemicals.	Heart muscle problems; anemia	Nausea, abdominal pain, diarrhea; hair and nail damage; fatigue; irritability.	Poultry, seafood; egg yolks; whole-grain breads and cereals; mushrooms, onions, garlic.
Copper	Component of several enzymes, including one needed to make body's pigments; stimulates iron absorption; needed to make red blood cells, connective tissue, nerve fibers.	In infants, anemia with abnormal development of bones, nerve tissue, lungs, skin and hair coloring.	Liver disease; vomiting; diarrhea.	Nuts; dried peas, beans; barley; prunes; organ meats; lobster.
Iodine	Essential for function of thyroid gland.	Goiter; delayed growth and development (cretinism) in infants.	Disturbed thyroid function; goiter.	Iodized salt; seafood; vegetables grown in iodine-rich soil.
Fluoride	Promotes strong teeth and bones, especially in children; enhances body's uptake of calcium.	Tooth decay.	Mottling of tooth enamel.	Fluoridated water; food cooked in fluoridated water; tea.
Manganese	Needed for healthy tendon and bone structure; component of several enzymes involved in metabolism.	Not known in humans.	Nerve damage.	Tea, coffee; bran; dried peas and beans; nuts.

form. First, the vitamin supplements available in pills are incomplete. Second, a pill results in a high concentration of vitamin that may interfere with the absorption of other nutrients from food. A diet based on the Food Guide Pyramid provides adequate amounts of all the vitamins, whereas indiscriminate use of supplements could result in toxic levels. Vitamin supplements should not be used except on the advice of your pediatrician.

Mineral	Effect	Signs of deficiency	Signs of overdose	Good sources
Molybdenum	Component of enzymes essential for metabolism; helps regulate iron storage.	Not known in humans.	Joint pain resembling gout.	Dried peas and beans; dark green leafy vegetables; organ meats; whole-grain breads and cereals.
Chromium	Works with insulin in glucose metabolism.	Symptoms resembling diabetes.	Not known for chromium in food; salts of chromium metal are toxic.	Whole-grain breads and cereals; brewer's yeast; peanuts.
Sulfur	Needed to make hair and nails; component of several amino acids.	Not known.	Not known for sulfur in food; salts of sulfur are toxic.	Wheat germ; dried peas and beans; beef; clams; peanuts.
Potassium	Works with sodium to regulate fluid balance; promotes transmission of nerve impulses and proper muscle function; essential for metabolism.	Muscle weakness; disturbances in heart rhythm; irritability.	Nausea, diarrhea; disturbances in heart rhythm that may lead to cardiac arrest.	Bananas; citrus fruits; dried fruits; deep yellow vegetables; potatoes; legumes; milk; bran cereal.
Sodium	Helps maintain fluid balance.	Rare, but loss of sodium can cause muscle cramps, weakness, headaches.	High blood pressure; kidney disease; heart failure.	Salt; processed foods; milk; water in some areas.
Chloride	Helps maintain acid-base balance of body fluids; component of hydrochloric acid in gastric juices needed for digestion.	Rare, but can upset acid-base and body fluids balance.	Upset in acid-base balance.	Same as sodium.

Minerals

Three minerals—calcium, phosphorus, and magnesium—account for 98 percent of the body's mineral content by weight. Calcium and phosphorus both play basic roles in countless biochemical reactions at the cellular level. They are also the main components of the skeleton.

Magnesium is a catalyst without which many metabolic functions could not take place.

Phosphorus is present in almost all animal and vegetable foods and usually occurs wherever calcium does. Milk and dairy products, fish bones (such as in canned salmon and sardines), and dark green leafy vegetables are the best sources of calcium. Magnesium, like phosphorus, occurs abundantly in animal and plant cells.

Both phosphorus and magnesium are easily absorbed and deficiencies do not occur in healthy children. By contrast, inadequate consumption of calcium is all too common, especially among adolescent girls who shun milk and dairy foods to avoid fat calories. These girls risk osteoporosis, or thinning of the bones, starting as early as age 30. Nonfat milk, yogurt, and other dairy foods are excellent sources of calcium and do not add unwanted fat calories to the diet.

The absorption of minerals is influenced by a number of factors, including certain hormones and vitamin levels. Infants absorb calcium more easily than adults do, and the rate of absorption is increased in the presence of other nutrients including the milk sugar lactose, the amino acids lysine and arginine, and vitamin C. Calcium absorption may be decreased by high dietary levels of phosphate, oxalate (in rhubarb and certain leafy green vegetables), or phytate compounds in fiber. Too much protein in the diet may increase the amount of calcium excreted in the urine.

Iron

Iron is a major constituent of hemoglobin, the red blood pigment that carries oxygen to the tissues. Lack of iron is the most common nutritional deficiency in the United States, and a frequent cause of anemia.

Babies are born with enough stored iron to last about 4 to 6 months. Pediatricians usually recommend an iron-fortified cereal when babies start solid foods, to prevent iron deficiency in the rapid growth phase of the first 2 years. Although cow's milk and breastmilk contain about the same amount of iron, a baby can absorb about 50

▷ **ELECTROLYTES**

The minerals potassium, sodium, and chloride are known as electrolytes. In the body, they conduct electrical currents and keep tissue fluids in balance, with positive potassium ions outside the cells, and positive sodium ions inside.

Potassium is essential to many functions, including the conduction of nerve impulses and muscle activity. A child may lose sodium and potassium through prolonged diarrhea, vomiting, or sweating, which lead to dehydration. Your pediatrician may recommend a commercial electrolyte solution to prevent serious electrolyte loss in a child with diarrhea or vomiting. For healthy children, fruits and vegetables are good sources of potassium.

Sodium and chloride combine to form sodium chloride, or table salt. These minerals are so plentiful in a normal diet, even without added salt, that deficiencies are seldom seen. Even though body reserves of sodium may be lost with prolonged diarrhea, vomiting, or sweating, it is almost never necessary to make up for sodium and chloride losses except by eating normal meals and drinking plenty of fluid. Salt pills can be dangerous for children and adolescents and should never be used.

percent of the iron from breastmilk compared with only about 10 percent of that in cow's milk. In addition, sensitivity to the protein in cow's milk can cause excessive iron loss through hidden bleeding from the digestive tract in babies under 12 months. This is why we recommend breastmilk or iron-enriched formula for children under one year. After age 2, the growth rate slows down, iron stores begin to build up again, and the risk of iron deficiency is much less.

Before adolescence, children normally take in adequate iron from a balanced diet that includes good iron sources, such as red meat and fortified cereals. In addition, fruits rich in vitamin C promote absorption of iron from plant foods. Adolescent boys may lack adequate iron around the peak growth period, when the iron stored in their bodies fails to meet the demands of rapid growth. Provided boys eat a balanced diet, the deficiency usually corrects itself after the growth spurt. Adolescent girls are at greater risk for developing iron deficiency anemia through loss of iron with menstrual blood, especially if they have heavy periods—a common occurrence in young women who have not yet established a regular pattern of ovulation. Girls who are menstruating should have a blood test for possible iron-deficiency anemia at every checkup.

Meat, poultry, fish and shellfish, legumes, and fortified cereals are good sources of iron. The amount of iron absorbed depends on the source. Iron from plant foods is absorbed least well; however, the amount can be increased by consuming foods with a high vitamin C content at the same meal. Tea, bran, and milk can inhibit the absorption of iron from plant foods. Absorption of iron from dairy foods is in the middle range, and the iron in meat is well absorbed.

Other Trace Minerals

Although required only in minuscule amounts, trace elements are involved in practically every process that takes place in the body. They are essential components of the enzyme systems that allow metabolic processes to take place. Without adequate levels, the body cannot maintain the proper fluid and chemical balances, or keep a steady heartbeat.

The 13 trace elements known to be nutritionally important are iron (see above), zinc, copper, fluoride, iodine, selenium, manganese, chromium, cobalt, molybdenum, nickel, silicon, and vanadium (for mineral requirements, functions, and sources, see pp. 100–102). Other minerals may also be required. Recommended dietary allowances have been established for four trace minerals—iron, zinc, iodine, and selenium—and safe and adequate amounts have been estimated for a further five—chromium, copper, manganese, molybdenum, and fluoride (for more about the importance of fluoride, see p. 35).

The body has a remarkable ability to regulate the balance of trace minerals. For example, if a person consumes more iron than necessary, the excess is usually excreted unchanged. However, if the body lacks iron, the rate of iron absorption from food is increased, to compensate. In rare cases, an inborn condition results in abnormalities of mineral absorption or storage.

Mineral deficiencies are not often seen in the United States, and children do not require mineral supplements unless they have a chronic condition that limits their diet or interferes with nutrient absorption. Therefore, iron, zinc, and other mineral supplements should never be given unless your pediatrician specifically recommends them.

Does my child have to eat each recommended serving from the Food Guide Pyramid every single day?
The Pyramid is a guide, not a prescription. It's not necessary to eat the exact number of servings from each group every day. Rather, intake should average out to the portions indicated over a period of 1 to 2 weeks, to ensure a healthy intake of calories along with all the essential nutrients. (See p. 89.)

The Food Guide Pyramid portions are very small. Do they really expect a hungry teenager to survive on half a cup of cooked pasta?
The portions are standardized to keep the Pyramid easy to use. Obviously, a person with a moderate appetite can eat much more than 1/2 cup of cooked pasta at a meal, and a single plateful may include several portions of one or several foods. Children's portions should be scaled according to age, appetite, and activity level (also see p. 92).

With all the concerns about fats, fiber, and obesity, should I just keep my children permanently on a no-fat, low-calorie, high-fiber diet?
Recommendations that children should eat only low-calorie, high-fiber foods are not to be trusted. A selection of foods from the Food Guide Pyramid every day ensures balanced nutrition. Children need calories for growth and activity, and some fat for health. And while fiber is good, too much of it could cause gas and other digestive problems and prevent a child from absorbing essential nutrients (see p. 91 for your child's recommended daily fiber intake).

CHAPTER 7

Spitting Up, Gagging, Vomiting, Diarrhea, and Constipation

Gail Laird panicked when her newborn, Owen, started spitting up cheesy white curds after every feeding. Responding to Gail's urgent call, her pediatrician calmed her fears. Owen wasn't really vomiting; he just opened his mouth and out came the milk. The baby was content and settling well both for his naps and at night, and the amount, when Gail really examined it, was tiny. The pediatrician assured Gail that Owen was fine, but asked her to call at once if the dribbling of milk ever changed to forceful vomiting and her baby was irritable or had other symptoms.

Most infants spit up small amounts of milk or formula during their first few months. Spitting up seldom indicates a medical problem or food sensitivity. In contrast to spitting up, vomiting involves forceful muscle contractions, brings up large amounts of milk, and distresses the baby and makes him uncomfortable.

The tendency to spit up decreases as the baby's gastrointestinal tract matures and usually stops altogether after he begins to sit. A few babies, however, continue to spit up until they are weaned to a cup or can walk on their own. (Also see Chapter 15.)

Gastroesophageal Reflux

Spitting up is sometimes associated with gastroesophageal reflux (doctors often refer to this as "GE reflux" or "GER" for short), which is usually a temporary mechanical hitch. If your baby's stomach is full or his position is changed abruptly after a feeding, the stomach contents—food mixed with stomach acid—press against the lower esophageal sphincter. This ring of muscle normally relaxes to let food pass from the esophagus into the stomach, then tightens again to keep the food there. When it is not fully developed, or it opens at the wrong time, the stomach contents flood back into the esophagus. In infants, gastroesophageal reflux rarely causes symptoms or distress and usually disappears as the lower esophageal sphincter grows stronger.

If your bottle-fed baby spits up unusually often, your pediatrician may recommend thickening his formula with a very small amount (1 to 3 teaspoons per ounce of formula) of rice cereal. Thicker liquid is more likely to remain in the stomach and reflux less easily. Never add solids to the bottle unless your pediatrician advises it. Unless carefully supervised, this practice not only may add unnecessary calories to your infant's diet, but also can interfere with the transition to solid foods (see Chapter 2). Your baby may also do better with smaller and more frequent feedings, but the total daily intake must be sufficient to keep up normal growth and development. You may find it helpful to keep your baby in an upright position in a stroller or carrier for the first hour or so after feeding.

In rare cases, gastroesophageal reflux is severe enough to cause symptoms such as bleeding, wheezing and hoarseness, or failure to gain weight. A baby with severe reflux may refuse to feed or be irritable after feeding. An older child may describe the discomfort typical of heartburn, and vomit or complain of a sour taste following regurgitation. These children need medical attention. Your pediatrician may prescribe treatment to lessen the secretion of stomach acid and help the muscle contract.

An older child with reflux should avoid fried and fatty foods because fat slows down the rate of stomach emptying and promotes reflux. Peppermint, caffeine (an ingredient of colas and many other soft drinks), and certain asthma medications can make the lower esophageal sphincter relax and allow stomach contents to flow back into the esophagus. Some experts believe that tomato-based products have a similar effect. If any food seems to affect your child adversely, keep it out of the diet for a week or two, then reintroduce it. If symptoms recur, avoid that food for a while.

Gagging

Every baby is born with the extrusion reflex, an automatic response that makes the baby push her tongue forward when an object is touched to it. As long as a strong extrusion response is present, a baby can't use the tongue to move food from the front to the back of the mouth in order to swallow. This is a mechanism that protects against potentially harmful material, including food a baby isn't ready to handle.

The extrusion reflex begins to fade when a child is about 4 months old. (In contrast, the gag reflex continues throughout life to protect against blockage of the airway.) This coincides neatly with the time when the baby doubles her birth weight and is beginning to need more nutrition

▶ **AIR SWALLOWING AND BURPING**

An infant who gulps down air with his breastmilk or formula is likely to spit up and burp more than others. It's usually possible to keep air swallowing (also called aerophagia) to a low level by feeding your baby as soon as he shows signs of being ready—before he starts to cry with hunger or frustration—and holding him at an angle to prevent air from entering his mouth as he feeds (also see Getting Started, p. 6).

Air swallowing and burping continue to occur in children long past infancy. Toddlers and older children swallow air when crying or when a stuffed-up nose makes them breathe through the mouth. Help your child to clear his nose frequently when a cold makes breathing difficult.

School-age children and adolescents gulp down air when eating or chewing gum; carbonated drinks also lead to gas buildup. Encourage your child to take a bit more time over meals and avoid carbonated drinks if gas is bothersome. For children who deliberately swallow air to gain attention with noisy belching, the best treatment is to let them know their behavior is unacceptable but avoid making it an attention-getting issue. Ignore it and eventually they'll stop because they are not arousing any reactions.

than breastmilk or formula provides (also see Chapter 2). Your baby will gradually learn to tolerate solids in her mouth as she sucks her fingers, toys, and other objects in her surroundings. It's not uncommon for babies to go through a stage of repeatedly gagging themselves with their fingers and even throwing up a bit. Some make a habit of this behavior after they are rewarded by a worried reaction from their parents the first few times. Eventually, a baby learns how far she can tolerate an object in her mouth and, at the same time, she improves her ability to swallow. This is all part of the complex process of learning to eat. Even after the early extrusion reflex has disappeared, a child will continue to gag from time to time when she has too much in her mouth, when she dislikes the taste or texture of a food, or when she feels pressured to eat.

Pouching

It's one thing to get food as far as a toddler's mouth, but it may be quite another to persuade her to swallow it. Toddlers and preschoolers are highly sensitive to tastes and textures. In addition, until about age 4, children don't develop the ability to chew efficiently with a grinding motion, which breaks food down to a manageable consistency. A strange food or too large a mouthful may trigger a fear of choking that makes a youngster reluctant to swallow. In particular, meat that has been chewed for a while can have a dry, pasty texture that makes young children gag.

Perhaps this is why toddlers very occasionally "pouch" their food, chewing it and wadding it in their cheeks. A poucher may carry food in his cheeks for hours, or leave a trail of chewed-up pellets in unexpected places. Pouching may be socially unacceptable, but it isn't a health hazard unless the wad is so large that the child could

 RUMINATION

In rare cases, a baby repeatedly gags, mouths, and reswallows regurgitated food to such an extent that his growth is impaired. This disorder, called rumination, is most likely to appear between ages 3 and 14 months, although older children may also be affected. It is more common in boys. Rumination is often associated with medical conditions such as severe reflux, emotional problems, and other factors affecting development. A child who is ruminating needs the attention of a pediatrician.

choke. It's not safe, however, to let a poucher nap or go to bed with food in his cheeks, because the wad could become dislodged during sleep and choke the child. If you can't persuade your child to spit the food out, try to clear the pouches with your finger. A child who keeps his teeth tightly clenched may open his mouth in spite of himself if you make faces with him in front of a mirror. Offer a drink of water to rinse out any remnants. (Also see p. 47.)

Pouching occurs infrequently and is a phase that will eventually pass on its own. However, you may be able to help it on its way if you:

- Present food in a form that your child enjoys chewing and swallowing.
- Offer alternatives if your child dislikes a particular food and is afraid of gagging.

For example, if meat is your youngster's stumbling block, make sure that the meat you offer is moist and easy to chew. Meat that's ground up and mixed with vegetables, such as in spaghetti sauce or chili con carne, is easier to manage than dry slices or grilled hamburger. In any case, meat isn't indispensable in the diet. Your child can obtain the same essential nutrients from other foods in the meat and protein group (see the Food Guide Pyramid, p. 90), such as fish, eggs, or dried beans and legumes, including peanut butter (thinly spread for children under age 4—and serve only smooth peanut butter to this age group).

A child who continues to pouch food after the early childhood years may be dealing with emotional stress. Your pediatrician will evaluate the child and recommend approaches to dealing with the condition.

Vomiting

An isolated incident of vomiting is nothing to worry about as long as your child is not unduly distressed and has no other symptoms such as a stomachache, earache, dizziness, diarrhea, or fever. In a baby up to 3 months, "fever" means a rectal temperature of 100.4°F (or 38°C), or higher; in all children over 3 months, it's a temperature of 101°F (38.3°C) or higher. If your child is older than 1 year, is eating and sleeping normally, and remains playful, you probably do not need to call your pediatrician. However, if your child has been vomiting persistently for 12 hours, has vomiting after a fall or head injury, or

◁ **DRINKS TO PREVENT DEHYDRATION IN A VOMITING CHILD**

For vomiting children, the main risk is water loss, or dehydration, especially if fever causes them to sweat more or they are also losing fluid through diarrhea. When vomiting is severe or prolonged, a child may become depleted of sodium, potassium, and chloride. These minerals have a crucial role in the transmission of nerve impulses and the contraction of muscles, and in regulating the body's fluid balance.

While missing a meal or two will cause no harm to an otherwise healthy child, it's important that a sick child continue to drink water to take care of normal daily needs, plus extra to make up for fluid loss and prevent dehydration. Infants and young children are especially susceptible to dehydration, as their kidneys are less efficient at conserving water than those of older children and adults. In addition, the small body size means that it takes relatively less fluid loss to lead to rapid dehydration.

Offer frequent sips of water or, if your child doesn't feel like drinking, ice chips to suck on. Build up to a fluid intake of 1 ounce an hour, then 2 ounces an hour until the child is able to drink normally.

Your pediatrician may recommend a commercial rehydration solution to help replace lost sodium and potassium in an infant or young child. Older children may ask for commercial sports drinks, but these should be used with care. They replace salts, but they also contain large amounts of sugar, which can make diarrhea worse. A child who wants a change from plain water may enjoy sips of fruit juice diluted half-and-half with water or flat soda pop. If your child is too sick to drink, call your pediatrician immediately.

A child who often feels nauseous and vomits when riding in cars, boats, or elevators suffers from motion sickness. The overwhelming nausea, vomiting, and headaches arise from a discrepancy between what the child can see and what she senses with the balance mechanism of her inner ear. If you're planning a trip by car, boat, or small plane, or know you'll be driving on winding roads, encourage your child to eat a light snack, such as a few crackers, before setting out. (She's more likely to feel sick if her stomach is either empty or overly full.) Make sure that her seat in the car or boat allows a clear view to the outside, preferably forward; many people feel less nauseous if they can focus on a point in the distance.

Some motion sickness sufferers find that chewing a few pieces of candied ginger helps to quell nausea, but the candy may be too spicy for a child's taste. Over-the-counter remedies can relieve the problem, although they also may cause drowsiness. Your pediatrician can advise you about preventive medications.

---

has associated symptoms, or if there's blood or greenish bile in the vomit, call your pediatrician immediately. Don't give anything to eat or drink until your pediatrician says it's safe. If your child is alert and complaining that she's thirsty, let her suck on ice chips or a frozen juice-pop to moisten her mouth and lips.

Similarly, if your infant's occasional vomiting or spitting up changes to forceful vomiting of fairly large amounts after every feeding, or if he is losing or failing to gain weight, call your pediatrician without delay. In a baby under 2 months of age, these symptoms may indicate pyloric stenosis, a narrowing of the passage between the stomach and the small intestine, or another condition requiring immediate treatment.

A child may vomit as a result of intense crying, particularly during a temper tantrum. Such tantrums are especially common between the ages of 18 months and 4 years, a period marked by opposition to parents and caregivers and conflicting feelings about increasing independence.

Vomiting or retching (dry vomiting) also may follow a coughing spell or accompany persistent postnasal drip. Emotional stress associated with major life changes, such as starting school or family upheavals, is a frequent cause of vomiting.

In most cases, the vomiting will disappear after the specific cause is identified and dealt with. Toddlers generally leave tantrums behind as they gain skills and enter the preschool years. (If a child continues to have frequent emotional outbursts after age 4, it may be advisable to ask your pediatrician for an evaluation and recommendations.) When a child has a cold, a good fluid intake is important to help thin secretions and clear mucus. When respiratory symptoms subside, vomiting associated with coughing and postnasal drip will decrease. A child who vomits in response to stress may continue to do so when faced with stressful situations. Your pediatrician can recommend behavioral measures to help the child cope with such challenges. In all cases, no special dietary measures are necessary. Your child

KEEP YOUR REGIONAL POISON CENTER'S PHONE NUMBER ON THE EMERGENCY LIST NEXT TO EVERY PHONE IN YOUR HOME.

■ A toddler or preschooler who vomits may have eaten or drunk something poisonous. If you suspect poisoning because of a telltale odor, burns or stains around the mouth, or an empty container, call the Poison Center immediately.

More than a million American children under age 6 suffer poisoning every year. Household cleaners, personal care products, and over-the-counter medications—including vitamins and iron supplements—lead the list of poisons.

Healthy preschoolers are both mobile and curious enough to sample even foul-tasting substances. To complicate matters, many caustic alkalis—such as drain cleaners, which can cause devastating injuries—have no taste. A child may ingest a large amount, therefore, before he or she stops because of a burning sensation. Vitamins, iron and other mineral supplements, and aspirin, while generally safe for adults, can cause serious or even life-threatening reactions in a child's small body.

■ Keep medications, personal hygiene products, and herbal and nutritional supplements locked up high out of the sight and reach of children.

■ Buy products with child-resistant caps and always replace the caps completely after use.

■ Never call medications "candy."

■ Empty and rinse all glasses immediately after gatherings where alcohol is served. Keep alcohol in a locked cabinet.

■ Lock cleaning products up high and out of reach, and never store cleaning products and other toxic substances in old food containers or other harmless-looking containers.

■ Keep a bottle of ipecac syrup in your home, but don't give it to your child unless your pediatrician or Poison Center says to do so. Ipecac, which induces vomiting, is not recommended for some poisons.

may resume normal meals as soon as he or she feels like eating again. (For the special problem of self-induced vomiting in adolescents who have serious eating disorders, see Chapter 10.)

A few children have periodic vomiting that occurs irregularly, without any warning symptoms, and lasts about 24 hours. During an attack, the child may feel lethargic and ill, but quickly recovers with no aftereffects and remains well until the next episode. This cyclic vomiting usually appears for the first time between 2 and 4 years. Attacks become less frequent and eventually stop as the child grows older. Migraine can also cause vomiting and abdominal pain. A child

It's usually unnecessary to give a vomiting child an antiemetic (a medication to suppress vomiting) because most vomiting in children results from a brief, self-limited viral infection of the gastrointestinal tract, or food poisoning.

Children may have severe vomiting, however, due to an ongoing medical condition such as complications of diabetes mellitus or treatment for cancer, or following anesthesia for surgery. In these cases, pediatricians prescribe antiemetics and other medications as necessary.

who has recurrent vomiting with or without headache or other symptoms should be evaluated by a pediatrician to identify possible triggering factors, such as food sensitivity, and to determine whether any treatment is required.

Diarrhea

Diarrhea is among the most common and recurrent childhood symptoms. Among children, diarrhea usually indicates acute infectious gastroenteritis, an inflammation of the lining of the digestive tract caused by a viral—or, less often, a bacterial—infection. In addition to loose stools, associated symptoms frequently include nausea, vomiting, and cramping. Outbreaks of infectious diarrhea occur frequently among youngsters in group childcare, especially at centers that care for children who aren't yet toilet trained.

While gastroenteritis itself is not a life-threat-ening infection, acute diarrhea can rapidly deplete a child's reserves of essential fluids and salts, particularly if he's also vomiting. Youngsters most at risk from the effects of diarrhea are those younger than 2, who are more rapidly susceptible to dehydration than older children and adults, and children with chronic illness, who are generally less able to ward off infection and compensate for the loss of fluids and nutrients.

Your pediatrician will advise you about giving your infant drinks to make up for the fluids and electrolytes (sodium, potassium, and chloride) lost with the diarrhea. Pharmacies and most supermarkets carry premixed drinks with the right balance of electrolytes. Homemade solutions should not be used. Drinks of clear liquids, such as juice, sport drinks, and soda pop, should not be given to infants.

On the other hand, an older child with diarrhea may drink clear liquids to make up for fluid loss. Clear broths and commercial rehydration solutions can help replace electrolytes. Sports drinks are best avoided because their sugar content can worsen the diarrhea and further injure the bowel. Resume small servings of a normal diet as soon as your child feels up to eating. Research has shown that with a normal diet, children main-

▷ **UNEXPLAINED VOMITING IN A TEENAGE GIRL**

An adolescent girl who is nauseated, faint, and vomiting for several days in a row may be pregnant or fearful that she is pregnant. If you have reason to believe she is sexually active and could be pregnant, discuss it with her calmly and consult your pediatrician without delay.

Injury to the bowel from infectious diarrhea may cause a temporary inability to digest lactose, the sugar in milk. A similar lactose intolerance can occur with antibiotic treatment. Until the tissues recover, the child cannot produce enough of the enzyme lactase to break down milk sugar. Consuming milk may result in the typical symptoms of lactose intolerance, including bloating, cramps, gassiness, and more diarrhea.

If your child wants milk or milk puddings, use only reduced-lactose milk for a week or two; aged cheeses, such as Cheddar and Parmesan, and yogurts are usually digestible because the lactose is broken down in the manufacturing process.

If symptoms are associated with antibiotic treatment, call your pediatrician, who may modify the prescription.

---

tain their weight better and may have diarrhea for a shorter time than when liquids alone are given. The BRAT (bananas, rice, apples, toast) diet, once recommended for convalescence from diarrhea, is no longer considered useful, and some pediatricians believe that it may actually prolong symptoms. The components of BRAT, however, will do no harm in a normal diet; bananas and cooked apples, in particular, have a binding effect, as do other fruits that contain high levels of the soluble fiber pectin. Oat bran is another excellent source of soluble fiber. Foods containing large amounts of insoluble fiber, such as wheat bran, promote bowel emptying and speed up bowel movements. They are best avoided until the bowel movements are back to normal.

Toddler Diarrhea

Ayesha's mother brought her 16-month-old in for a consultation: "Ayesha has terrible diarrhea—five or six movements every day, and they're very liquid," the mother related. "Not only that, but she's losing everything she eats. I can see whole pieces of vegetables and other foods in her diapers. I'm afraid she's not getting enough nourishment."

A quick review of the records showed that Ayesha was growing and gaining weight satisfactorily. She was an active, adventurous toddler, making enthusiastic efforts to speak, and eating well, though with a toddler's typically limited attention span.

While in the pediatrician's office, Ayesha demanded, "Drink juice!" Her mother pulled a bottle of apple juice out of her shoulder bag.

"This is all she'll drink, Doctor. She practically lives on juice."

In reality, the juice was probably responsible for Ayesha's loose stools. A toddler may have several loose bowel movements every day, passing fairly large fragments of undigested food together with a lot of liquid. Parents worry that the child has something wrong with his bowels and is not absorbing his food properly. This nonspecific diarrhea is common among toddlers and is not a cause for concern provided the child is active, healthy, and gaining weight. Toddlers eventually grow out of this phase. When a cause can be found, it's often too much fruit juice in the diet. Toddlers love to drink sweet juice and parents give it to them, thinking it's nourishing.

In fact, juice has several strikes against it. First, it contains large amounts of several sugars, including fructose and sorbitol, which can lead to loose stools. Apple, pear, grape, cherry, and prune juices, among others, have a high sorbitol content. (Sorbitol, often used to sweeten "sugarless" candies and gums, cannot be digested. It's not unusual for children to develop diarrhea with gassiness and bloating if they frequently chew sugarless gum.) Second, toddlers tend to fill up on juice and don't have enough room left for more nourishing foods at mealtimes. Third, juice is not an important source of nutrients. It's true that citrus juices and those fortified with vitamin C are good sources of this vitamin, but there's no reason to overdo the recommended daily serving of one-fourth to one-third cup (2 to 3 ounces) for a toddler. Finally, the sugar in juice can harm developing teeth if a toddler has free access, such as in a bottle that she carries about with her. When you serve juice, serve it in a cup at a scheduled snack or meal. If your toddler is thirsty, she'll find water more thirst-quenching than sugary juice. Developing a preference for water may also

 OTC MEDICATIONS

> Over-the-counter antidiarrheal medications are not recommended for children aged 2 years and younger and should be used only on a pediatrician's advice in older children. These medications cause fluid and salt to stay in the intestine, which appears to stop the diarrhea. In fact, they may make it more difficult to recognize dehydration.

help to eliminate a source of unnecessary calories in the future.

Diarrhea caused by bacteria (for example, salmonella or shigella) is of special concern among children of all ages, especially in schools and group childcare. If your infant younger than 3 months has diarrhea and a fever, call your pediatrician right away.

If your baby is older than 3 months and has diarrhea and a mild fever for more than a day, check whether she's passing a normal amount of

 ROTAVIRUS: A COMMON CAUSE OF WINTERTIME DIARRHEA

In the United States, rotavirus accounts for about 20 percent of all cases of childhood gastroenteritis, and is the most common reason that young children are hospitalized for dehydration. The effects can be serious: Rotavirus infection is implicated in approximately 100 childhood deaths from diarrhea each year. Like the viruses for influenza and the common cold, rotavirus is most active in the winter and spring—October through May—though infection can occur at any time of the year. Vaccines are currently under development. Until they become available, simple hygiene is the best defense. Parents and others involved in children's care must not only wash their own hands but also continually teach youngsters how important it is to wash hands before handling food and after using the toilet in order to restrict the spread of this and other sicknesses.

Recent outbreaks of serious food poisoning have been traced to *Escherichia coli (E. coli)* O157:H7. This microbe is a rogue strain of the bacterium *E. coli*, which normally lives in human and animal digestive tracts and helps keep harmful germs from invading the body and causing illness. Strain O157:H7 produces toxins that cause severe, bloody diarrhea and may lead to fatal kidney failure (hemolytic uremic syndrome, or HUS).

The most common source of illness is undercooked ground beef from packing plants that prepare meat in bulk for fast-food chains. *E. coli* O157:H7 has also been found in roast beef, raw (unpasteurized) milk, contaminated water, and vegetables contaminated with cow manure. People have become ill after drinking unpasteurized cider made from unwashed apples contaminated with cow manure. The bacteria can be passed from one person to another or through cross-contamination of foods. (Several other foodborne parasites are causing new health problems; see Chapter 13.) Though *E. coli* O157:H7 survives freezing and can multiply at low temperatures, it is destroyed by thorough cooking.

To reduce your family's risk of foodborne illness, follow these safety rules (also see p. 173):

- Bag meats separately from other foods at the supermarket.

- Don't allow juices from meat to mix with other foods.

- Follow safe-handling labels on meat and poultry.

- Refrigerate meat at 40°F or freeze immediately.

- Use separate cutting boards for meat and produce.

- Wash cutting boards with hot soapy water and disinfect with a solution of 1 part bleach to 10 parts water before using again.

- Wash and disinfect knives and other utensils that have touched raw meat.

- Cook hamburger until brown in the center and the juices run clear. Ground beef is safely cooked when it reaches an internal temperature of at least 160°F. Reheat ground-beef leftovers to 165°F.

- Larger cuts of beef may be eaten medium to rare provided they have reached an internal temperature of at least 140°F. Use a meat thermometer if you find it hard to judge when meat is done.

- Wash fruits and vegetables.

- Don't let your youngsters sample uncooked dough or batter made with raw eggs. Use only commercial mayonnaise, and don't use raw eggs in uncooked desserts (such as frozen meringue made with whipped egg whites).

urine, check her temperature with a thermometer, then call your pediatrician.

If an older child has diarrhea lasting longer than 48 hours, vomiting longer than 12 hours, or associated symptoms such as headache or blood in the stool, call your pediatrician.

The dietary recommendations for managing bacterial diarrhea are similar to those for viral gastroenteritis (see p. 114). An infant should continue with breastfeeding or formula; your pediatrician will advise whether additional fluids are necessary. An older child should drink plenty of clear fluids to keep tissues hydrated. Drinks with a high sugar content, such as undiluted fruit juices and sports drinks, may worsen the diarrhea. Juices should be diluted half-and-half with water. As soon as the child feels well enough, she should resume small servings of a normal diet. If symptoms recur when your child drinks milk, switch to reduced-lactose or lactose-free milk for about 2 weeks. Cheese and yogurt are usually digestible (see Temporary Lactose Intolerance Following Diarrhea or Antibiotic Use, p. 114).

Intestinal Disorders

Jeffrey, at 7, had a nagging, recurrent stomachache that was making it difficult for him to go to school. He had no other symptoms, such as vomiting, fever, or headache, but the stomachache was severe and sometimes made him double over in pain. His parents, enmeshed in a bitter and complicated divorce since Jeffrey was 5, at least shared concern over Jeffrey's health. They appeared at the pediatrician's office together.

The pediatrician soon saw that the parents had called only a limited truce. When the doctor asked how the pain began, Jeffrey's mother explained, "It started the day my son's Dad introduced him to his new girlfriend—"

Jeffrey's father cut in. "You know it started that day I dropped Jeffrey off and you lost control. You used bad language in front of my son and called me terrible names."

Jeffrey's physical examination was normal, but the child seemed anxious and sad. The pediatrician told his parents that there was nothing wrong with Jeffrey's stomach. Rather, his heart and mind had too much to bear and the emotional overload was causing Jeffrey's pain. He referred the parents to a counselor to help Jeffrey over the long term, and scheduled a follow-up appointment to see Jeffrey in a month.

IRRITABLE BOWEL SYNDROME. Starting in the school years, many young people are troubled by a condition known as irritable bowel syndrome (IBS) or spastic colon. Typical symptoms are irregular, alternating cycles of constipation and diarrhea accompanied by pain or cramping, gas, and bloating. Although uncomfortable during the daytime, the symptoms do not waken the child at night. Irritable bowel syndrome symptoms don't have a consistent trigger, although anxiety plays a role and attacks may be more intense at times of stress, such as school tests or family upheaval. Food sensitivity may be a cause in some cases, but true allergy is not a factor. The condition runs in families; often, one parent also has IBS.

Irritable bowel syndrome is not a serious disorder and it doesn't lead to more serious conditions. While the symptoms are uncomfortable, they are not associated with weight loss, fever, or abnormalities in any specific laboratory test. However, because all the symptoms of IBS may mimic potentially serious diseases, a child with recurrent bowel upsets should be evaluated by a pediatrician to rule out other conditions, such as inflammatory bowel disease.

A child with IBS should consume plenty of sol-

Inflammatory bowel disease (IBD) is a term that includes ileitis (Crohn disease) and colitis. Whatever the specific diagnosis may be, symptoms include severe diarrhea, blood and/or mucus in the stools, pain, weight loss, recurrent fever, mouth sores, and joint pain. When the onset is in childhood, inflammatory bowel disease may impair growth and delay sexual maturation. In fact, in some children impaired growth becomes a problem before any bowel symptoms appear.

Diarrhea associated with bowel inflammation often leads to malnutrition, because the absorption of nutrients is impaired. In addition to a generalized malnutrition, young people with IBD suffer from specific problems depending on the site of inflammation in the bowel. Children with IBD may need more calories than healthy children to make up for the losses due to illness. Unfortunately, the child may have a poor appetite and fear that eating will make symptoms worse.

The immune system and certain infectious organisms are thought to contribute to the development of IBD. No specific foods have been found to worsen symptoms. Therefore, there's no reason to restrict the diet unless a child dislikes certain foods or believes they worsen symptoms.

uble fiber. Excellent sources are oat bran, vegetables, and fruits, which contain pectin. Your pediatrician may recommend behavioral approaches for managing stress. Occasionally, medications are prescribed.

MALABSORPTION. Several conditions may hinder the absorption of nutrients in the small intestine. Such malabsorption disorders may involve one or several nutrients, and the diagnosis depends on the type and number of nutrients that are lacking. Irrespective of the diagnosis, the general symptoms are similar: irritability, diarrhea, weight loss, bloating, and gas. The stools are often bulky and unusually foul-smelling. They may also be pale and float on the water surface because of a high fat content.

Less severe malabsorption syndromes, such as lactose intolerance (see following section), can be managed by reducing or eliminating one specific nutrient and finding substitutes. Youngsters with more severe disorders may suffer malnutrition not only because they don't absorb essential nutrients but also because they often feel too poorly to eat and they need more calories than they can consume. A child with symptoms suggesting a malabsorption disorder should be seen promptly by a pediatrician, who will perform diagnostic tests to identify the cause. Depending on the diagnosis, the child may be referred for specialist consultation; an expert pediatric dietitian must assist with dietary planning.

LACTOSE INTOLERANCE. Lactose intolerance is perhaps the most widely known malabsorption state. Transmitted genetically, it is most prevalent among people of African, Asian, and Native American ancestry, and is relatively uncommon among those of Northern European descent. The symptoms of lactose intolerance usually appear at about age 3 or 4, when the child gradually stops producing lactase, the enzyme essential for the digestion of lactose, the sugar in cow's milk. Typical symptoms—cramps, gas, and diarrhea—follow the consumption of dairy products. Lactose intolerance is rare in very young children, except after a gastrointestinal illnes or antibiotic treatment. When it occurs, typical symptoms are irritability, gas, and diarrhea.

Babies with lactose intolerance should drink formulas based on milk substitutes. Older children and adults are advised to keep to a lactose-free diet that eliminates most milk and dairy foods. Many children with lactose intolerance are also intolerant of soy products. Parents and children alike must become expert label-readers, to identify terms that indicate the presence of milk and other foods linked to intolerance. There are many people, however, who have only a partial intolerance and can handle milk and dairy products so long as small amounts are served as part of a meal. Aged cheeses and yogurts are usually acceptable because lactose is broken down in the manufacturing process. Reduced-lactose milk is widely available, as are lactase enzyme preparations that can be added to milk and dairy foods to make lactose digestible. However, in the rare cases where milk and dairy products have to be avoided altogether, it's essential to provide alternative sources of calcium, such as canned fish with bones (sardines, salmon, herring, mackerel), tofu, broccoli, and other high-calcium foods. Your pediatrician may recommend a calcium supplement.

GLUTEN ENTEROPATHY. People with gluten enteropathy or celiac disease cannot tolerate gliadin, a protein constituent of gluten, which is found in many grains. The symptoms of gluten enteropathy usually appear after a baby is first given cereal containing wheat, oats, barley, rye, buckwheat, or millet. Affected children are irritable; they grow and gain weight poorly. They often have diarrhea, although some may be constipated. This food intolerance is fairly rare and can be difficult to diagnose. It tends to run in families and is most common in those of European and Middle Eastern descent. Treatment requires strict, lifelong avoidance of cereals, pasta, breads, and baked goods made with grains containing gluten. Also banned are commercially produced foods such as canned soups and stews thickened with processed grains and cereals. Your pediatrician will provide dietary advice and refer you to a nutritionist for guidance with your child's diet.

CYSTIC FIBROSIS. Cystic fibrosis (CF) is an inherited condition that affects the function of every organ but especially the glands that produce mucus in the lungs, pancreas, liver, and

▷ **HIRSCHSPRUNG DISEASE**

If your new baby has only rare bowel movements, her stools are hard, and her abdomen appears bloated, your pediatrician will examine her to determine whether retained stool is distending the abdomen while the rectum is empty. This group of symptoms can indicate Hirschsprung disease, a rare condition in which the baby lacks the nerves needed for having bowel movements. Hirschsprung disease is treated with surgery. Left untreated, it can lead to life-threatening complications, so be sure to bring early constipation to your pediatrician's attention.

intestines. Mucus blocks the ducts in the pancreas and interferes with the secretion of enzymes and juices that are essential for digestion. Although young people with CF may eat large amounts, they often become malnourished because they cannot absorb nutrients. The stools of those with CF are pale, bulky, and fatty.

The severity of CF varies widely. Each child's diet must be individually prescribed and monitored to compensate for specific nutrient losses as well as to make sure the child consumes enough calories. Many children with CF need supplementary enzymes to compensate for damage to the pancreas. Children with CF lose excessive amounts of sodium and chloride in their perspiration and thus need additional salt during hot weather, when they have a fever, or in other conditions that cause them to sweat a great deal. Selenium supplements, once promoted as a miracle cure, have not been found to help those with CF.

Constipation

Constipation is among the symptoms pediatricians are asked about most often. People have the

▷ **DEALING WITH STOOL RETENTION**

Stool retention is fairly common among school-age children. What happens is that the child repeatedly ignores the urge to move his bowels. The nerve sensations in the area gradually grow weaker, and the intestine is less able to contract. The impacted stools become progressively larger, harder, and more painful to pass. This, in turn, makes the child even more reluctant to have a bowel movement. Eventually, liquid stool may leak out around the mass of impacted stool, staining the underwear and bedsheets. The child isn't aware that he's passing the liquid stool, and the parents are misled into thinking he has diarrhea. When the pediatrician examines the child, however, the true problem becomes apparent.

Don't try to treat constipation or stool retention yourself with over-the-counter laxatives or enemas. Whatever the reason for stool retention may be, your child needs a pediatrician's help to overcome it. The goals of treatment are the following: (1) to set regular bowel habits; (2) to recognize and respond to the urge to defecate; (3) to hold stool only until the time and place are right for a bowel movement; (4) to focus the family's attention away from the child's bowels; and (5) to eat foods that help keep bowel movements regular.

Treatment usually starts with medication to help the child pass the impacted feces and thus let the bowel shrink back to normal size. Then the child continues taking a daily dose of a medication to ease stool passage. The pediatrician keeps a close check on the child's diet to make sure he's consuming plenty of fluids together with fiber in the form of vegetables, fruits, and whole-grain cereals and breads. Treatment may take a long time and involve the whole family. Relapses are not uncommon, but the problem usually will resolve.

Adolescents with bulimia—the binge-purge syndrome—frequently abuse laxatives to provoke diarrhea and purge unwanted calories. Constipation, by contrast, is a recognized complication of anorexia nervosa (also see Chapter 10). Apart from a diet that is woefully deficient in nutrients and bulk, the anorexic has weakening of the intestinal muscles and an overall slowing of body metabolism, both of which are directly due to starvation. In addition, adolescents with this serious eating disorder typically drink very little for fear of becoming bloated. The weight of stool retained in the intestines can make it difficult to judge whether treatment is progressing. Finally, constipation may be worsened by medications used to treat anorexia.

Specialists treating adolescents with anorexia manage constipation by providing a diet that includes adequate fiber and fluids. Moderate exercise is encouraged. Stool softeners and other medications are used if necessary.

idea that constipation means not having a daily bowel movement. Many parents think their children will get sick if they don't have a movement every day. This isn't so. Some children (and adults) have several bowel movements every day, while others go two or three days or even longer, then pass a stool of normal consistency. A person is constipated only when the stool is hard or dry and can't be passed without straining or causing pain. Constipation may occur when the diet is lacking in fiber and fluid or when a child has been inactive and has taken fluids poorly during a viral illness.

It's quite normal for a breastfed baby to pass stools only once every two or three days, or even less frequently. This is because babies digest their mothers' milk so completely that there's not much residue. In contrast, some babies may pass stools several times a day, whether on breastmilk, formula, or a combination. This, too, is normal. As long as your baby is gaining weight and the stools are soft—semiliquid and seedy in a breastfed baby, no firmer than peanut butter in a for-

mula-fed infant—the bowel movements are normal. If your baby's stools are hard and dry, like marbles, or watery and filled with mucus, or whitish and claylike, talk to your pediatrician.

Occasionally, an infant becomes constipated with the introduction of solid foods between 4 and 6 months, or when cow's milk is introduced to the diet after about 1 year. If your pediatrician suspects that constipation is making your bottle-fed baby younger than 4 months irritable and uncomfortable, he or she may recommend adding $1/2$ to 1 teaspoon of dark sugar syrup or malt extract to each of four formula bottles per

▷ DON'T GIVE LAXATIVES OR ENEMAS

Never give laxatives or enemas to treat your child's constipation unless your pediatrician prescribes them. Used improperly, these products can disrupt bowel function and worsen the problem.

day for 2 to 4 days. If treatment is necessary for your infant between 4 and 12 months, your pediatrician will advise you. It often helps to give the baby a small amount of diluted apple juice or prune juice, or a few teaspoons of puréed prunes. Changing from rice cereal to oatmeal to increase the intake of soluble fiber can help to clear up the problem. "Loosening" foods, such as puréed apricots, may help. In addition, a small serving ($1/4$ to $1/3$ cup) of prune or pear juice may have a laxative effect. Foods that tend to make stools firmer, such as bananas and applesauce, should be reduced or avoided until the problem is resolved.

A lot can be learned from vegetarians. They are rarely constipated because their diet includes a large amount of fiber. To keep your children's bowel movements regular, make sure their meals and snacks include high-fiber foods such as fruits, vegetables, and whole-grain breads and cereals. Nutrition experts recommend as a general rule that a person's daily intake of fiber should equal his or her age plus 5 grams (thus, for a 7-year-old, 7 + 5 = 12 grams a day) up to a maximum of 35 grams a day. Oat bran cereal and popcorn are good sources of fiber that many youngsters like to eat. A couple of prunes or a small glass of prune juice can help stimulate bowel function. Prunes contain a natural laxative, called isatin, as well as lots of soluble fiber and sorbitol—a naturally occurring, nonabsorbable sugar alcohol—both of which have laxative effects. Apple juice and pear juice are also good sources of sorbitol; however, cooked apples, such as in applesauce, may contribute to constipation and are often given to help children with the opposite problem: diarrhea. Plenty of water—6 to 8 glasses a day—is needed to help dietary fiber do its job. Finally, regular exercise helps promote regular bowel function.

When Constipation Looks Like Diarrhea

A few days before a long-planned family vacation, Carol Larson urgently had to talk to her pediatrician. "We're supposed to catch a plane next weekend and Brendan has diarrhea." she said. "If I bring him over to your office, will you give him something so we can get through this?"

When the pediatrician examined 5-year-old Brendan, he found no sign of diarrhea, but he saw loose feces smeared on the child's underwear. This led the doctor to question Brendan and his mother about the child's usual bowel habits.

Brendan, it turned out, had very irregular bowel movements and was afraid to use the toilet. He often appeared to be trying to hold back a bowel movement. On the rare occasions when he couldn't hold it back, he would demand a diaper. His mother could hear the child crying and straining behind the bathroom door. Finally, Brendan would emerge and give the diaper, soiled with loose stool, back to his mother, and the cycle would begin all over again.

The pediatrician explained to Carol that Brendan didn't have diarrhea. On the contrary, the child had severe constipation as a result of withholding stool. Liquid stool leaking out around an impaction—a large amount of stool in the colon—gave the appearance of diarrhea.

The doctor outlined a treatment plan to help Brendan overcome his stool retention and fear of using the toilet. The first step was to empty the rectum of hard stool. An enema cleared out enough of the impaction so that Brendan and his family could leave as planned, and the child would have only a minimum amount of loose fecal overflow during the week's vacation. After they returned, a regular program including stool softeners and changes in toileting procedures solved the problem. It took several weeks, however, to change these habits.

My mother-in-law says my baby isn't getting enough to eat because he spits up a lot. She says if I would just add some cereal to his bottle, he wouldn't spit up.
Spitting up is normal and rarely interferes with a baby's nutrition. If your baby spits up unusually often, your pediatrician may recommend thickening his formula with a very small amount of rice cereal. Never add solids to the bottle unless your pediatrician advises it. The baby also may do better with smaller and more frequent feedings (see p. 107).

My 8-year-old has terrible gas. He embarrasses me by burping loudly when we go out.
School-age children and adolescents gulp down air when eating or chewing gum; carbonated drinks also lead to gas buildup. Encourage your child to take a bit more time over meals and to avoid carbonated drinks if gas is bothersome. If he belches noisily to gain attention, let him know this behavior is unacceptable but avoid reacting with the extra notice he craves (see p. 108).

My toddler wads up food in his cheeks. Is this behavior a health hazard?
Pouching isn't a health hazard unless the wad is so large that the child could choke. It's not safe, however, to let a poucher nap or go to bed with food in his cheeks. If you can't persuade your child to spit it out, try to clear the pouches with your finger and give him a drink of water to rinse his mouth (see p. 109).

My daughter dreads long car trips because they make her sick to her stomach. I tried a medication from the pharmacy, but it made her sleepy.
Encourage your child to eat a few crackers or another light snack before setting out. Make sure that her seat allows a clear view to the outside; many people feel less nauseous if they can focus on a point in the distance. Your pediatrician will advise about preventive medications (see p. 111).

How long should I keep my child on a soft diet when he has diarrhea?
Resume small servings of a normal diet as soon as the child feels up to eating. Bowel movements return to normal faster with a regular diet than when only soft foods are given (see p. 114).

Can irritable bowel syndrome lead to serious diseases like cancer?
Irritable bowel syndrome does not lead to more serious conditions. However, because all the symptoms of irritable bowel syndrome also may be associated with potentially serious diseases, a youngster with recurrent bowel upsets should be evaluated by a pediatrician, to rule out other conditions (see p. 117).

CHAPTER 8

Is My Child Too Fat?

Most parents are happy if their children have outstanding talent, looks, intelligence, or athletic ability. Size, however, is a different story. They prefer that their children blend in with the crowd, neither much smaller nor much larger than others the same age. That was why Bill and Judy brought their 8-year-old daughter, Letitia, for an evaluation. Letitia's height of 48 inches was nothing out of the ordinary, but at 75 pounds, she was heavier than 90 percent of girls her age. Always plump, Letitia had become notice-ably overweight in the past few months. Her parents, who were of average build, insisted that Letitia "hardly ate a thing." They were concerned that a glandular problem might be causing their daughter to gain weight.

It had been a year and a half since Letitia's last checkup, and her health—apart from the worry over her weight—was good. The family had moved to the community within the year and they had only just gotten around to finding a pediatri-cian. According to Bill and Judy, the weight gain had started during this time. The chart from Letitia's former pediatrician backed them up.

Letitia had no signs of the rare medical prob-lems that might cause weight gain in a school-age child. Careful probing by her pediatrician uncov-ered the source of the problem. She was unhappy about the move and slow to make friends. She wasn't involved in sports or hobbies and spent all her spare time watching television. The lack of

In the United States, at least one child in five is overweight, and the rate is growing. Over the past two decades, the number of overweight children has increased by more than 50 percent and the number of extremely overweight children has nearly doubled.

physical activity and the constant snacking that went with TV watching had contributed to her weight gain. Her parents were aware that Letitia was having problems adjusting, although they hadn't linked such problems with the excessive weight gain. They saw that she was not eating much at meals, but they weren't aware of how many high-calorie snacks Letitia put away after school at the neighbor's house where she stayed until her parents came home from work. Letitia didn't have a glandular problem and she didn't need a formal weight-loss program. She simply needed to get away from the TV and overeating, and develop interests that would keep her active and help her make friends.

At their pediatrician's suggestion, Bill and Judy enrolled Letitia in after-school swimming classes at the local boys' and girls' club. A new sitter, who walked Letitia to and from the club, made sure that snacks included fruit, raw vegetables, and low-fat dips and yogurt. Letitia's growth contin-ued, but with the exercise and more healthful eat-ing, a slim, fit Letitia began to emerge out of her cocoon of overweight and inactivity. She found friends among her fellow swimmers and gradu-ally shed her homesickness.

Why Do Children Become Overweight?
Children become overweight for many reasons. A tendency to be overweight may run in some fami-

lies. Many children don't get enough physical activity. Some young people develop unhealthy eating patterns, possibly because they copy examples they see at the family table. In most cases, overweight is probably a combination of factors. Medical problems, such as hormone imbalances, are rare, and account for fewer than 1 out of 100 cases of childhood obesity. Children with rare, severe metabolic disorders such as Cushing syndrome, Prader-Willi syndrome, and Turner syndrome may have problems with hearing, vision, and development in addition to overweight and short stature. Such conditions are usually diagnosed early in life. A pediatrician will perform a physical exam and diagnostic tests in the unlikely event that he or she suspects problems of this type.

Although weight problems run in families, not all children with a family history of obesity will be overweight. If parents' weights are normal, slightly overweight children between the ages of 1 and 3 do not have an increased risk for overweight later in life. However, children whose parents or brothers and sisters are overweight have a higher risk of becoming overweight themselves. While genetic factors play a role, a shared environment also influences body weight. For example, some children overeat because their parents habitually overeat and unwittingly encourage the children to do the same.

Passive relaxation, such as watching TV for hours on end as Letitia did, is probably a major factor in the rising tide of childhood obesity. Snacking while watching TV adds to the problem. Children who watch more than 5 hours of television a day are 4.5 times more likely to become overweight than those who watch for 2

▷ **FAT AND HAPPY? MAYBE NOT**

Apart from the health problems linked to overweight in children, there are also psychological and social consequences, especially if overweight continues into adulthood. Some studies have shown that children as young as 6 may associate overweight with negative stereotypes. Asked to rank drawings of children, youngsters deemed overweight children less likable than those who had various physical handicaps. Overweight children are often less likely to be chosen for team activities and may have more difficulty in making friends. Because overweight children are bigger than others their age, people tend to overestimate how old they are and expect them to reach unreasonably high standards of behavior and achievement. To avoid the teasing of their own age group, some overweight children turn to younger children for friendship. Furthermore, overweight children often have trouble finding clothes that fit in styles they like. Ultimately, overweight adolescents may develop a distorted body image, which puts them at risk for eating disorders.

Studies have shown that being overweight weakens the chance of being accepted into a high-ranking college and reduces a job applicant's attractiveness to prospective employers. Overweight can translate into lower social and economic levels and, for women, less likelihood of finding a mate. Negative perceptions about weight are directly and indirectly passed on to children; thus, the consequences of overweight are carried on.

> Dr. Dietz's law of energy consumption: Children use up more energy doing almost anything besides watching TV.

hours or less. If your youngster is spending too much time in front of the box, turn it off. Keep snacks for snacktimes, such as after an outdoor game, not as an accompaniment to TV.

As with other issues, children's perceptions about weight are influenced by the views of their parents and peers. When Jim and Linda brought their 11-year old son, Evan, to see his pediatrician, it was clear that Jim, a fit runner, was extremely concerned. Asked to rate Evan's weight problem on a 10-point scale, Jim gave it a 10, but when Linda was asked to do the same, she scored it as 2. Evan was caught in the middle. Though he hadn't been bothered by his weight before, his father's attention had made it an issue. Yet his mother's apparent lack of concern sent Evan a confusing signal. An easygoing boy, he wanted to please both his parents and wasn't sure how to do so.

Their pediatrician showed the family where Evan ranked in the weight and growth charts. He explained that it wasn't unusual for boys to gain several pounds, as Evan had, with the hormonal changes leading up to puberty. In most cases, they lose this extra weight as they enter the adolescent growth spurt. Evan wasn't seriously overweight; however, a program begun now to promote weight control, healthy eating, and fitness could prevent his fleshiness from developing into flab. The pediatrician advised the family, however, that such a plan could succeed only if everyone agreed on a common goal and how best to reach it.

It's essential to find out how an overweight child perceives his weight and whether he wants to do something about it. A weight-management program is doomed from the start if *only* the parents *or* the child perceives a problem that requires action. Without this agreement, conflicts and resentments are likely to prevail when one side advocates weight loss and the other resists.

Is My Child Too Fat?

Pediatricians evaluate children's growth and build by means of standardized growth charts (see Appendix III) and body mass index (BMI, Appendix IV). The growth charts show whether a child falls within the normal range of height and weight for her age. Children with weight or height above the 95th or below the 5th percentile should be examined with special concern about whether further evaluation is needed.

Body mass index is a calculation of your child's weight relative to height. A BMI above the

▷ **CHOOSE TO BE HAPPY**

> Many adolescents, particularly girls, become deeply unhappy when they realize that they are never going to be shaped like supermodels or earn multi–million-dollar contracts as movie stars.
>
> Help your daughter to feel comfortable with who she is. Reassure her that real beauty is more than skin deep. Offer her role models among women who have made the most of their talents, achieving intellectual and humanitarian goals, or raising healthy, balanced children, instead of trading on their looks for superficial success.

85th percentile indicates overweight, above the 95th, severe overweight. Revised charts to identify percentiles will be available in 1999 (see p. 221).

Growth charts and BMI tell only part of the story, however, because neither method measures body fat. The results can be misleading for those with unusually muscular or lean builds. It's possible to have a high BMI without having excess fat. In some obesity clinics, as many as 10 to 15 percent of children are in this category. To determine if a child is carrying too much fat, doctors use skinfold calipers—an instrument that looks like a pair of spring-loaded tongs—to gently pinch the flesh on the trunk and the back of the upper arm. The results, based on resistance to the pressure exerted by the calipers, indicate how much fat lies directly under the skin. This method measures body fat directly, so frame size and muscle mass don't interfere with the accuracy of the measurement. If there is excess fat on these sites, it's safe to assume there's excess fat elsewhere. However, if a child's weight for height is above the 95th percentile while her skinfold measurements are normal, she is considered to have a large frame but not too much fat.

If this is the case with your child, reassure her that her extra weight is not fat and encourage her to be physically active to maintain her muscle tone. Be sure to include yourself in any discussions with your pediatrician about your child's weight. To prevent worries about body size, both parent and child need to accept the child's body type. Other members of the family may have a similar build. If you focus inappropriately on

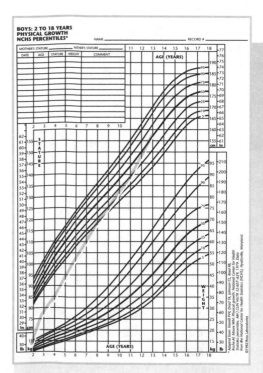

SHORT AND STOCKY
BIRTHWEIGHT: 8 POUNDS 0 OUNCES
LENGTH AT BIRTH: 21 INCHES
HEALTH: EXCELLENT
PARENTS: MOTHER 5' 2", 120 POUNDS
FATHER 5' 8", 175 POUNDS

This boy was born normal weight and length to parents who were slightly shorter than average. Although he stayed within the normal range for height and weight until about age 8, his weight gain accelerated until, by age 13, he was well outside the normal range of weight for height. His pediatrician recommended that the family seek help from a nutritionist who specialized in weight management for adolescents in order to prevent further weight gain and give him time for his height to "catch up" to his weight.

TALL AND SLENDER

BIRTHWEIGHT: 10 POUNDS 12 OUNCES
LENGTH AT BIRTH: 22 INCHES
HEALTH: EXCELLENT
PARENTS: MOTHER 5' 11", 150 POUNDS
FATHER 6' 5", 200 POUNDS

This girl was born large and has remained outside the normal range for height and weight. Although at age 3 her weight is outside the normal range, she is not overfat and her weight is in proportion to her height. Because her parents are tall, chances are she will continue to be taller than most children her age.

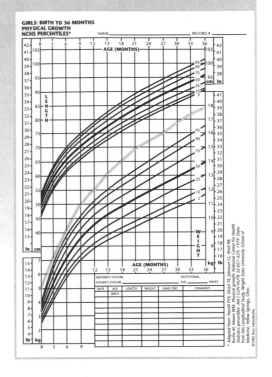

weight alone and pester your child to lose weight, she may develop a distorted body image and risk an eating disorder (see Chapter 10). It's estimated that 70 percent to 80 percent of girls perceive themselves, whether rightly or wrongly, as fat.

Experts warn that a misperception of body image may be partly fueling the current obesity epidemic, with inappropriate dieting followed by rebound weight gain.

The case histories reported here illustrate how individual growth problems might be handled.

Making a Change for the Better

If your pediatrician recommends a weight-management plan, it's important to find the best way to help your child learn to control his weight and prevent a problem that could carry over into adulthood.

Involving the whole family in weight control encourages healthful habits without singling out the overweight child. Children are quick learners and they learn best by example. If you eat a variety of foods and are physically active, you will teach your children healthy habits they can follow for the rest of their lives. How you manage the changes that need to be made depends largely on your child's age. A 6-year-old, for example, doesn't need lengthy explanations; just make the changes that are in her best interest. A 10-year-old, however, may be more cooperative if he understands the reasons for change: "We're having turkey tonight instead of hamburgers because it's lower in fat. And that's good for us," or, "You had cake—lots of calories—today at the birthday party, so tonight we're having fruit for dessert— no fat and plenty of fiber and vitamins."

Teenagers may resist being told what to do,

even though they need direction. Giving unsolicited advice may be asking for trouble; rather, pick your moments carefully. If your teenage daughter wails, "I'm fat!" it's your chance to ask, "Is something bothering you? Is there some way I can help?" But try not to seem overly eager or the window of opportunity may be slammed shut. Here are some other helpful tips:

BE A GUIDE, NOT A DICTATOR. Provide a variety of healthful foods and help your children learn how to choose wisely for themselves: what to eat and how much. The more you push a child to eat a particular food, the more likely she is to resist. On the other hand, forbidden foods—as by the edict "No candy, ever!"—may seem especially desirable.

DON'T LIMIT YOUR CHILD'S CALORIES. Your child should never be on a calorie-restricted diet unless your pediatrician prescribes and closely supervises it. Limiting what children eat can deprive them of essential nutrients and interfere with growth and development.

CUT DOWN ON FAT IN YOUR FAMILY'S DIET. Reducing the fat in your family's diet is the first step toward preventing excess weight gain in children. In any case, for long-term health, children older than 2 should take in no more than 30 percent of their total daily calories as fat, with one-third or less (10 percent of calories) as saturated fat. Simple fat-cutting steps include serving low-fat or nonfat dairy products, lean meats and skinless poultry, fish or occasional vegetarian entrées, and low-fat or fat-free breads and cereals. If you plan a major dietary overhaul, you may benefit from the advice of a registered dietitian (RD); ask your pediatrician for a referral.

REMEMBER THAT A CALORIE IS A CALORIE, WHEREVER IT COMES FROM. Even reduced-fat foods can be high in calories because of their simple sugar content and other ingredients. Although you should not be counting every calorie your child eats or restricting calories, allowing unlimited access to many "diet" foods can lead to undesirable weight gain.

ALLOW A TREAT ONCE IN A WHILE. Occasional treats of ice cream, potato chips, candy, and the like do no harm. Banning them outright may make them seem overly desirable.

AVOID TEMPTATION. Free access to a supply of cookies, candy, and other treat foods will sabotage efforts to moderate your child's food intake. Buy or make what you need for a special occasion, but don't keep such foods on hand.

LIMIT TAKE-OUT AND FAST FOODS. Products tend to be high in fat and the portions are over-large.

WHENEVER POSSIBLE, PREPARE MEALS AT HOME AND INVOLVE CHILDREN IN THE PREPARATION. It's easier to control the fat content and portion sizes of foods prepared from healthful raw ingredients in your own kitchen. Children may be more likely to eat food that they help buy and prepare.

OFFER WATER FOR DRINKS, RATHER THAN JUICE OR SODA POP. Water does not promote weight gain and is better for children's teeth than a sugary bath of juice or soft drink.

MAKE SURE THAT YOUR CHILD CONSUMES 24 OUNCES (THREE LARGE GLASSES) OF SKIM OR LOW-FAT MILK, OR THE EQUIVALENT IN OTHER DAIRY FOODS, PER DAY. Milk and dairy products are the best sources of calcium, which is essential for strong bones, teeth, and a healthy body. Girls, in particular, need calcium, but may skimp unless persuaded that consuming good calcium sources will not lead to weight gain.

ENCOURAGE CHILDREN TO EAT SLOWLY. Your child will be better able to judge when she has eaten enough if she eats at a moderate rate and does not rush her food.

KEEP A PLACE FOR EATING AND KEEP EATING IN ITS PLACE. Allow eating only in designated areas, such as the dining room or kitchen. Keep mealtimes calm and sociable without distractions such as TV. Serve meals and snacks on a regular, but not inflexible, schedule.

INVOLVE CHILDREN IN FOOD SHOPPING AND MEAL PREPARATION. Grocery shopping with your child is an opportunity to pass along nutrition lessons, such as comparing the labels on sugared and nonsugared cereals for calories, sodium, and price per serving. Some markets have candy-free check-out lines. When shopping with children, avoid the check-out line with a candy display.

STAY FLEXIBLE. New issues arise as a child becomes more independent, and family and school schedules change. Any change that takes place after the initial treatment plan has begun will require a rethinking of your current weight management techniques.

Healthful Choices

As a parent, you determine what food is offered and when. Your child decides whether and how much to eat. That's why you should offer healthful choices. Let your child choose between an apple and air-popped popcorn for a snack, not an apple or a chocolate-covered cookie. You create an atmosphere for lifelong healthy eating when children are allowed choices and not dictated to. Above all, don't ask your child what he or she wants to eat unless you are prepared to serve it. Refer to the Food Guide Pyramid (p. 90) for guidelines regarding balanced nutrition and age-appropriate serving sizes.

Be consistent. You inadvertently reinforce undesirable behavior—such as demands for candy at the check-out counter—by inconsistently "giving in" to it. When you allow treats for

▷ **LET GROWTH CATCH UP**

The goal for overweight children between ages 2 and 7 is weight maintenance, not to reduce weight. For a heavy but otherwise healthy child, it's more important to develop habits of healthful eating and activity. If an overweight child maintains her weight as she grows, her weight and height will come back in proportion and her BMI will drop.

parties or other special occasions, make it clear that these are exceptions.

Make any change with the idea that it's permanent, and not just a temporary fix. A healthy approach to eating and physical activity should become your lifestyle, rather than a patch over a weight problem.

Changes in diet and activity are easier to take if they are made gradually. Try only one or two changes a week and stick with them. Here are a few examples of small changes that make a big difference over time:

▷ For children older than 2, switch from whole milk to low-fat or fat-free milk. Serve reduced-fat cheese and nonfat yogurt. Fat should not be restricted from the diets of children under age 2, because it is needed for proper brain growth and development.

▷ Go for family after-dinner walks.

▷ Keep unsalted pretzels on hand for snacks.

▷ Switch from full-fat bread spreads, such as mayonnaise and dressings, to reduced-fat or fat-free varieties. There are plenty of brands to choose from. Make sandwiches with reduced-fat spreads.

▶ Substitute low-fat sandwich meats such as turkey bologna and turkey ham for beef and pork products. Use ground turkey instead of beef for pasta sauces, chili and tacos, and casseroles.

▶ Serve frozen juice and fruit bars without fat or added sugar, instead of ice cream. Frozen yogurt, even if promoted as a low-fat or fat-free dessert, may be high in sugar and, therefore, in calories.

▶ Serve low-fat popcorn instead of cookies for after-school snacks.

▶ Naturally low-fat cookies, such as vanilla wafers, graham crackers, and gingersnaps, are good choices for cookie fans, but if there is a favorite that your child just can't do without, find or make a low-fat version of it.

▶ Make gravies and sauces virtually fat-free by reducing defatted broth or vegetable stock with seasonings.

▶ Experiment with child-friendly vegetarian recipes such as spaghetti or lasagne made with vegetables instead of meat, together with reduced-fat cheeses.

Getting Expert Help for Weight Management

If you find changing your family's eating habits too difficult to do alone, you could benefit from outside help. Start with your pediatrician. He or she may refer you to a registered dietitian who specializes in children's nutrition and can help develop a plan tailored to your family's lifestyle and preferences. However, if more intense efforts are needed or your pediatrician warns that your child's health is at risk unless she loses weight, you may need to consider a formal treatment program. A university-based medical center should be able to help you find a pediatric weight-control program suitable for your child. Contact the Weight-Control Information Network (WIN) for information (1 WIN Way

Bethesda, MD 20892-3665; Phone (301) 984-7378 or (800) 946-8098; E-mail: win@info. niddk.nih.gov; Internet: http://www.niddk.nih.gov/health/nutrit/win.htm.

A child experiencing sleep apnea (interrupted breathing during sleep), a child younger than age 2 who is severely overweight, or a child older than 2 whose BMI is above the 99th percentile should be evaluated in a pediatric obesity center before a weight control program is considered.

If your older child is not ready to change or your family is not committed to helping, a weight management program is a waste of time and may actually be harmful. A failed weight-control program can diminish a child's already low self-esteem and hinder future efforts at weight control. Moreover, if the child is depressed or has an eating disorder (see Chapter 10), she requires psychological evaluation and treatment in addition to weight control. A depressed, overweight child may have sleep disturbances, feelings of hopelessness and sadness, and appetite changes. A therapist may recommend counseling before, or along with, a weight management program.

For older children, outside help may be essential. Take Liz, for example. Every time her mother cautiously touched on the topic of Liz's growing weight, the 15-year-old burst into tears. Liz knew she had a problem, but took her mother's unsolicited advice as a criticism of her personality. Confrontations ended with raised voices and slammed doors. Liz's mother backed off and made the wise decision to bring the girl in to see her pediatrician, with whom Liz felt comfortable. After listening to both sides, her doctor found that mother and daughter were in agreement. He referred Liz and her mother to a dietitian who specialized in working with overweight adolescents, and suggested Liz call for a follow-up appointment when she had been in a weight-management program for 3 months.

Weight-Loss Programs

Commercial weight-loss programs generally are not designed with children or adolescents in mind. However, some new programs do address children's problems. As you evaluate a program, go through this check list:

✔ **Is it staffed with a variety of health professionals?** The best programs include one or more registered dietitians or qualified nutritionists, exercise physiologists, pediatricians or family physicians, and psychiatrists or psychologists.

✔ **Does the program focus on behavioral changes?** This includes how to select healthful foods in appropriate portions, or how to exercise more while limiting sedentary behavior.

✔ **Does it include a medical evaluation?** Before your child is enrolled in a program, her weight, growth, and general health should be reviewed by a pediatrician. In addition, a health professional should monitor the child's weight, growth, and general health at regular intervals during the course of the program.

✔ **Does the program encompass the whole family and not just the overweight child?**

✔ **Is the program appropriate for your child's age and capabilities?** A program for 8- to 12-year-olds, for example, differs from programs for 13- to 18-year-olds in terms of the responsibilities placed on the child and the parents.

✔ **Does the program include a maintenance program?** Support and referral resources are essential for reinforcing behavior and dealing with the underlying issues that led to overweight.

Numerous camps offer weight-control programs for young people. One advantage of such

▷ **A FAMILY AFFAIR**

Children younger than 10 whose parents are overweight are more than twice as likely to become overweight adults as children the same age but with normal-weight parents.

places is that all the campers are overweight and the fear of being teased or stigmatized is less. But like other marketed weight-loss programs, they have a high relapse rate.

Getting Active

Children are increasingly overweight because, although they eat no more than youngsters did 20 years ago, by most accounts they are less active. One survey has found that fewer than 25 percent of children in grades 4 through 12 take part in 20 minutes of vigorous activity or 30 minutes of any physical activity every day. For fitness, experts recommend at least 30 minutes of activity most days of the week. Budget restrictions force many schools to limit physical education, but children shouldn't depend on organized sports for exercise. Unstructured outdoor play is a good outlet for energy. City parents may have to make a special effort to find places where children can play freely; even some suburban parents are concerned about letting young children play outside without adult supervision. Following are some tips for becoming more active:

▷ **Be a role model.** If your children see that you are active and enjoying it, they are more likely to be active and stay active into adulthood.

▷ **Walk more.** If you live close enough, encourage your children to walk to school with friends, or walk with them.

▶ **Limit sedentary activities.** The American Academy of Pediatrics recommends a daily limit of no more than 1 to 2 hours for watching television and videos or playing computer and video games. (Only nonviolent games should be chosen.)

▶ **Help your child find physical activities.** Be sensitive to your child's needs; overweight children often feel self-conscious about taking part in sports. Look for activities that your child enjoys and that aren't embarrassing or too difficult.

▶ **Provide toys and gear that make your child want to become active.** For example, give a gift of tennis or riding lessons, along with the appropriate gear.

▶ **Offer activities, not food, as rewards.** For example, go bowling for a treat rather than staying home to make double hot-fudge sundaes.

▶ **Push your local school board to make physical education a priority.** Also push for healthy choices in vending machines. Get involved with the parent-teacher organization to see that school meals and snacks offer varied, healthful, and low-fat food choices.

▶ **Volunteer to help out with school or community sports programs.** If you're involved in the school's extracurricular activities, your child is more likely to take part.

▶ **Plan activity parties.** For example, invite neighborhood youngsters to a backyard hula hoop tournament.

▶ **Check out biking and hiking trails.** Then take the family for weekend outings.

▶ **Recruit your children to clean the car,** instead of going to a car wash.

▶ **Go on a mall walk** (but steer clear of the food court) or collect a library of child-friendly exercise videos and exercise along with your child.

Team sports such as soccer, basketball, volleyball, hockey, lacrosse, and football are excellent outlets for energy. For children who dislike team sports, swimming, skating, dance classes, gymnastics, and martial arts are among the many excellent alternatives.

Family Involvement

If parents are overweight, it's unlikely that a child's weight problem can be successfully addressed unless the parents' lifestyle and eating habits are revised as well. That's another reason parents should take part in their child's weight-control program. If your child is the only family member who has to change his eating and exercise habits, he may feel resentful and is likely to relapse. On the other hand, slender siblings may chafe if they perceive that limits are placed on their foods and activities for the sake of one family member's weight problem. Encourage youngsters to express their feelings openly. Answer their objections truthfully and fairly. Above all, try to prevent destructive sarcasm and teasing by family members or others from sabotaging serious efforts at weight control.

The chances of long-term success are better if all caregivers, including baby-sitters, childcare center staff, and grandparents are aware of the plan and accept responsibility to help the overweight child in her efforts while respecting her evolving independence.

ISSUES PARENTS OFTEN RAISE ABOUT CHILDREN'S WEIGHT

Those really overweight children usually have glandular problems, don't they?

Medical problems linked to overweight are rare, accounting for fewer than 1 out of 100 cases of obesity in children. Many factors, such as overeating, inactivity, and parents' behavior, contribute to the rising tide of overweight among children in this country. (For more about this, turn to p. 125.)

I think my 12-year-old son is getting pudgy and needs to go on a diet. His mother says I'm making a fuss about nothing.

It's not unusual for a boy to gain several pounds with the hormonal changes leading up to puberty. In most cases, the extra weight drops off during the adolescent growth spurt. To settle the argu-

ment, ask your pediatrician to check where your son fits on the standard growth chart. This will help you plan a weight-management strategy, if one is needed. Join your son in healthy eating and exercise to control his weight and get fit (see pp. 127 and 129).

My daughter and I agree that she needs to lose weight. I've just started a low-calorie diet, so it'll keep things simple if she does the same, won't it?

Your child should not be on a calorie-restricted diet unless your pediatrician prescribes and closely supervises it. Limiting what children eat can deprive them of nutrients and interfere with their growth and development. (For suggestions on how to approach weight problems in children, turn to p. 130.)

CHAPTER 9

Is My Child Too Thin?
Too Small? Too Tall?

Although overweight is the more common problem, some parents worry because their children appear too thin. At age 11, Eric was 58 inches tall and weighed only 60 pounds. His parents, Paul and Cindy, couldn't help noticing Eric was by far the thinnest child in his class, and he seemed to look even skinnier as he grew. Paul and Cindy had no worries about Eric's eating habits and he seemed healthy and energetic, but they kept bringing up his weight at each of Eric's checkups. Their pediatrician confirmed that while Eric's height was average, he was thinner than most boys his age, falling within the 5th percentile according to the growth charts (see Appendix III). Nevertheless, he assured them that Eric was a healthy boy. A check of the family history revealed that in college, Paul had never weighed more than 150 pounds, although his height was 6 feet 2 inches. He had gained a few pounds in the intervening decades, but was proud that he could still wear the suit he was married in 15 years before. Their pediatrician suggested they stop worrying about Eric's weight. Thinness, he said, was "in the genes," and Eric's build was lean and wiry, like his dad's.

Parents concerned about a child's weight are doing the right thing by bringing him to the pediatrician's office for evaluation. In most cases, the child's weight is within normal range and the child is growing normally. However, a sudden change in the rate of growth or a loss of, or failure to gain, weight may signal a developing problem.

That was the case with 15-year-old Sandy. Her parents, Sharon and Bill, had noticed that their usually healthy teenager seemed fatigued and frequently complained of gas, bloating, and crampy diarrhea. One day Sharon was startled to see that Sandy's jeans and skirts suddenly looked too big for her. At first, they simply chalked the changes up to her incredibly busy schedule and irregular eating habits. But when Sandy told them she had lost 10 pounds in the last two months, they made an appointment with their pediatrician. Sharon and Bill were shocked when their doctor told them tests had confirmed his suspicions: Sandy had Crohn disease, an inflammation of the intestinal tract. Because this chronic condition interferes with the absorption of nutrients, it can cause weight loss in a fully grown adolescent, as Sandy was, or hinder growth and weight gain in a younger child. In severe cases, a youngster may become undernourished. Sandy received intensive outpatient treat-

At regular examinations, beginning with the first one after birth, your pediatrician keeps track of your child's weight and height. During the first two years, the head circumference is also routinely measured as an index of growth and development. Chronic illnesses can slow growth. Such illnesses sometimes occur silently, with no apparent symptoms. That's one of the reasons that regular checkups are important for your child's health.

Occasionally, parents consult their pediatrician because their child is taller and thinner than others the same age. If the pediatrician finds that the child is unusually tall and slender for his or her age, with noticeably long, thin, loose-jointed limbs, fingers, and toes, tests may be ordered to rule out Marfan syndrome. This rare inborn condition can cause heart problems in addition to skeletal and eye abnormalities. It requires the attention of a specialist.

ment to stabilize her condition. Crohn disease is a lifelong condition that Sandy will have to manage with nutritional and medical treatments as necessary. Her parents acted wisely in consulting their pediatrician as soon as they suspected something was wrong. In this way, they may have prevented Sandy from becoming severely ill.

Tracking Your Child's Growth

The most dramatic growth spurts occur during the first year of life and later with the onset of puberty. A healthy infant may double his birth weight by four months and triple it by the first birthday. The intensive growth of the first 12 months is followed by a relative slowing of the growth rate, accompanied by a noticeable drop in the child's appetite during the second year—a turn of events that can be disturbing to parents, at least with the first child. Because children tend to grow in spurts, a marked gain in height may be followed by a period when height slows a bit and weight catches up, or vice versa. The appetite varies according to the rate

of growth and the amount of energy the child uses. This cycle of feasting and fasting recurs to some degree throughout childhood, and weight gain is continuous but not always steady. Normal fluctuations in appetite do not affect your child's overall rate of growth.

In an infant younger than 1 year, a marked drop-off in weight gain or growth rate could signal a feeding or developmental problem, or a medical condition such as failure to thrive (FTT). This is a potentially serious condition, the causes of which are often difficult to pinpoint. A pediatrician may suspect failure to thrive if a baby falls below the 5th percentile for height and weight. An older child should be checked by his pediatrician if height falls off but weight gain continues.

The last dramatic growth spurt occurs during adolescence, when boys may sprout up as much as 4 inches a year and girls grow and mature seemingly overnight. For the pediatrician assessing your child's height and weight, an unexplained major change or lack of change over time is more important than any single measurement. If your daughter has not shown signs of puberty

At about 6 months, babies who are exclusively breastfed may have a drop-off of weight relative to length, which continues to increase. In fact, the baby's rate of growth may cross growth-chart percentiles. However, this normal slowing of weight gain is no cause for concern so long as the child continues to grow steadily in length.

(breast enlargement, growth of pubic hair, menarche or first period) by age 13, or your son has no corresponding signs (growth of pubic and body hair, enlargement of sexual organs) by age 14, consult your pediatrician.

Growth Charts: By the Numbers

Normal children come in a dazzling variety of shapes and sizes, and the rates of growth and weight gain vary widely. A group of 8-year-olds, for example, may vary by as much as 30 pounds in weight and 8 inches in height without being considered abnormally tall, short, heavy, or thin, as long as their individual heights and weights are in proportion. Pediatricians use standardized growth charts like those in Appendix III to determine whether children fall within the normal range, and track each child's growth rate over time. Typically, pediatricians weigh and measure children at regular visits every 6 months up to age 2, then once a year after that. Heights and weights marked on charts provide a picture of the growth pattern.

Weight or height alone doesn't tell the whole story; a child's weight in relation to height is what counts. Another method increasingly used to determine whether a child has a normal weight for his height is the body mass index (BMI), a calculation based on height and weight (see Appendix IV). A BMI above the 95th percentile is unusually high and suggests the child may have a weight problem. (See Chapter 8 for more about overweight.)

How Much Is in the Genes?

Both height and weight tend to run in families, and you can get a rough idea of how tall a child is likely to be by looking at the parents. Here's one way to predict a child's probable height at maturity: Add together the heights of the mother and father in inches and divide by two. For a boy,

 GROWTH PROBLEMS IN ADOPTED CHILDREN

Occasionally, children adopted from other countries may have slow growth and developmental delays as a result of inadequate care and nutrition. These young people may need special help and more calories than usual to catch up to a level appropriate for their age. Adoption agencies can put parents in touch with support groups for those in similar situations. Your pediatrician will help with advice and referrals to specialist care, if required.

add 2 1/2 inches; for a girl, subtract 2 1/2 inches. Though this is just a rough estimate, it provides a guideline. Quite simply, the taller the parents, the taller the child is likely to be, while short parents tend to have short children.

The same holds true for build. As with Eric, whose lean frame resembled his father's, a child's build often reflects that of his parents. Studies with twins have confirmed this genetic connection, but environment, too, can play an influential role. A child may have a genetic predisposition to thinness—with thin parents, siblings, and even grandparents—but if the diet he is offered includes large amounts of high-fat, high-calorie foods and he spends most of his time watching TV or playing computer games, his environment may overpower his genes and he is at risk for becoming overweight.

If Your Child Is Unusually Short or Tall

Such is the value placed on height in our society that once children reach school age, parents worry if their otherwise healthy son looks considerably shorter than other boys his age, though they are generally less concerned if he is unusually tall. Girls who are short tend to elicit less attention. In most cases, short children are simply following their genetic pattern.

In rare cases, children fail to grow because they are deficient in growth hormone, which is produced by the pituitary gland. When a growth hormone deficiency is present, regular injections of human growth hormone 3 to 7 days a week over a period of 4 to 5 years may help some children grow. However, a medical study has called into question the overall effectiveness of this treatment. Pediatricians do not advise treating a healthy, short child with growth hormone just to make him conform to some arbitrary notion of desirable height. The question of treatment should be discussed with a pediatric endocrinologist—a doctor who specializes in hormonal functions in children and who can best judge whether your child might benefit from growth hormone. If you are undecided or feel you don't have enough information, seek a second opinion. Growth hormone treatment has risks and side effects, and may cost thousands of dollars a year. Many health insurance plans do not pay for growth hormone treatment unless a deficiency is present. If your child has a proven deficiency and growth hormone is prescribed, therapy should begin as early as possible, because treatment produces faster and greater growth when given to younger rather than older children.

The long-term risks of human growth hormone treatment are not yet known. However, while one purpose of giving growth hormone is to improve a child's self-image and enable him to fit in with others his age, the need for injections over a period of years may only reinforce the negative self-image that already overshadows many of these children.

Rarely, when a child is abnormally tall, the cause may be a tumor of the pituitary gland that releases excessive amounts of growth hormone. This stimulates growth, particularly of the jaw and the long bones in the arms and legs. Disproportionate height cannot be reversed, but the condition can be treated with surgery, medications, or irradiation.

Finally, some children are born small because of intrauterine growth retardation, and they never catch up. A baby may be abnormally small for many reasons, including a decreased blood supply to the placenta; exposure to infection, drugs, or alcohol while in the womb; a chromosomal disorder; or extreme prematurity. For these children, small size is normal. They should not be overfed or given growth hormone to add either pounds or inches.

Although genes influence a child's growth potential, the size of a baby born after a full-term pregnancy with no medical problems has little or no relationship to his size at maturity. Most children grow and gain weight rapidly for their first 6 to 12 months. However, parents are taken by surprise when the growth rate suddenly slows at about 1 year and the child's appetite also falls off to compensate for a corresponding decrease in energy requirements. This phase, which many pediatricians refer to as "catch-down growth," is a normal development. Parents of toddlers typically worry that their child isn't eating enough when this drop-off of appetite occurs. Provided the child continues to grow and gain weight steadily but more gradually, there is no cause for concern. Pushing him to eat will not increase his appetite or his growth, and may foster resistance. Some examples of children and their growth patterns show what varying growth rates can mean.

NORMALLY SMALL

BIRTH WEIGHT: 9 POUNDS 2 OUNCES

LENGTH AT BIRTH: 19 INCHES

HEALTH: EXCELLENT

PARENTS: MOTHER 5' 1", 100 POUNDS

FATHER 5' 6", 145 POUNDS

Although this girl's weight at 24 months falls below the "normal" range, her weight is in proportion to her length, which is also below the 5th percentile. Because both parents are small, for this child, this is a normal rate of growth.

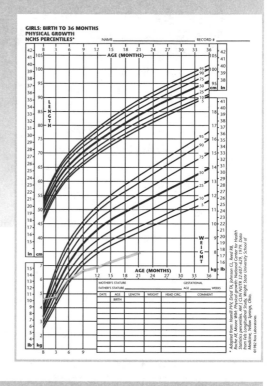

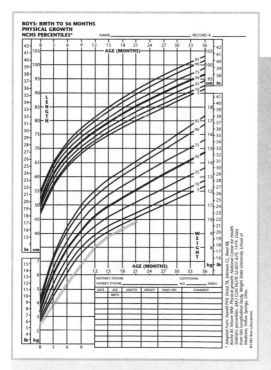

FETAL ALCOHOL SYNDROME

BIRTH WEIGHT: 5 POUNDS 0 OUNCES

LENGTH AT BIRTH: 18 INCHES

**HEALTH: DIAGNOSED WITH FETAL ALCOHOL
        SYNDROME**

PARENTS: MOTHER 5' 5", 130 POUNDS

FATHER 6' 0", 180 POUNDS

Fetal alcohol syndrome, the result of excessive alcohol intake by the mother during pregnancy, retards growth during pregnancy (intrauterine growth retardation). Although this boy's weight is in proportion to his length at 21 months, his length is below the 5th percentile and his growth followed the curve shown here. He falls outside the normal range for both weight and length and is unlikely ever to catch up.

NORMALLY THIN

BIRTH WEIGHT: 7 POUNDS 5 OUNCES
LENGTH AT BIRTH: 21 INCHES
HEALTH: EXCELLENT
PARENTS: MOTHER 5' 4", 135 POUNDS
FATHER 5' 10", 175 POUNDS

Although this boy's birth weight was average, his weight shifted to well below average by the time he was 24 months old, and he appeared quite thin. His length was normal. While neither parent is thin, a medical history revealed that the child's father weighed only 130 pounds in high school, although he had already reached his current height. Considering the leanness of his father as an adolescent, the child's weight, which is in proportion to his height, is appropriate.

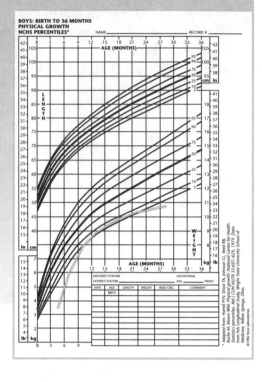

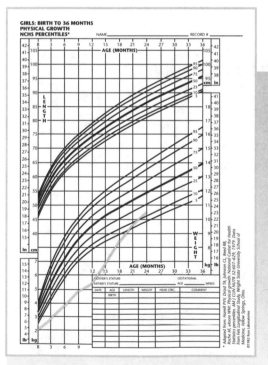

PREMATURE BIRTH

BIRTH WEIGHT: 4 POUNDS 2 OUNCES
LENGTH AT BIRTH: 17 1/2 INCHES
HEALTH: BORN AT 30 WEEKS, BUT HEALTH IS GOOD
PARENTS: MOTHER 5' 7", 140 POUNDS
FATHER 6' 2", 190 POUNDS

Because this girl was born 8 weeks premature, she started out small, but her length and weight were proportionate to each other. If you take into account the fact that she was born early and backtrack 8 weeks on the growth chart, it puts her well within the normal range of height and weight. As with most pre-emies, her growth and weight gain had entered the normal range by her second birthday.

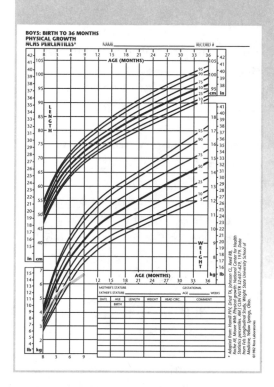

UNEXPLAINED CHANGE

BIRTH WEIGHT: 8 POUNDS 0 OUNCES

LENGTH AT BIRTH: 20¹/₂ INCHES

HEALTH: EXCELLENT

PARENTS: MOTHER 5' 10", 145 POUNDS

FATHER 6' 0", 175 POUNDS

This boy was born with normal weight and length and seemed to be progressing normally for the first few months. Between 6 and 9 months, however, both weight and height fell below the normal range. Because he started out normally but his growth then suddenly dropped off, he should have a complete medical examination.

NORMALLY LARGE

BIRTH WEIGHT: 6 POUNDS 5 OUNCES

LENGTH AT BIRTH: 17 INCHES

HEALTH: EXCELLENT

PARENTS: MOTHER 5' 6", 150 POUNDS

FATHER 6' 3", 245 POUNDS

This girl was born small. However, both parents have large frames and are muscular. Her father was a football player in high school and college. During the girl's first three years, she began to catch up to her genetic potential and developed a large frame. She was overweight for her height, but her skinfold measurements showed she was not excessively fat. There is no reason to be concerned about her size.

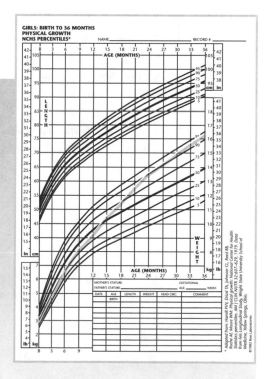

My child is noticeably taller than all the other children in his grade. Most people tell him he's lucky being very tall instead of short, but I wonder if his unusual height could be a signal that something is not quite right.
If you have any concerns at all about your child's growth, arrange a consultation with your pediatrician, who will examine your child and perform any tests that may be necessary. In most cases, there's nothing to worry about. For the pediatrician assessing your child's height and weight, an explained major change or lack of change over time is more important than any single measurement (see p. 138).

My daughter was premature and although she eventually caught up in development, she has remained very small in comparison to other girls in her class. Could growth hormone treatment help her catch up in size?
For a child born very prematurely, such as your daughter, small size may be normal .

She should not be given growth hormone or extra calories to add pounds or inches. Help her understand that her height is what's right for her, and to feel comfortable with herself (p. 140).

When should my baby double his birth weight?
A healthy infant may double his birth weight by 4 months and triple it by the first birthday. However, these are only guidelines. Every child grows at his own rate, which is not necessarily identical to that of others the same age (see p. 138).

How can I tell if my child is growing at an acceptable rate?
At every examination beginning with the first one after birth, your pediatrician will check your child's height and weight and compare these measurements with standard growth charts. For the first 2 years, your pediatrician will also measure your baby's head circumference as an index of growth and development (see p. 137).

CHAPTER 10

Eating Disorders

Kathleen, at 16, regularly brought home excellent school reports and was a dedicated ballet student. Her parents were understandably very proud of her accomplishments.

Although she had many friends and an active social life, some girls resented the way their parents cited Kathleen as an example: "Why can't you be more like Kathleen? She's so smart and her mom tells me she works very hard. She never talks back to her parents, and she's almost certain to get into a good college."

Knowledgeable about food, Kathleen sometimes prepared elaborate dishes for special occasions. However, she was usually too busy to join the family at the table, and often declined to eat with the excuse that she felt full after picking at food on the run.

Odd behaviors and rituals involving food are common in children and adolescents. In most cases, they fade away over time and have no adverse effects on health. Eating disorders, by contrast, are persistent patterns of behavior that are associated with psychological issues, lead to serious health problems, and can endanger life.

When she did eat with the family, she took tiny portions, cut them into ever-diminishing pieces, and never finished a plateful. The increasingly rare family meals began to turn into pitched battles, with Kathleen's mother urging her to eat and her father trying to make peace between them. As soon as the table was cleared, Kathleen rushed off to the ballet barre in her room, where her parents could hear her exercising for hours, even late at night.

It was the ballet teacher who brought up the idea that Kathleen's behavior might be more than adolescent obstinacy: "Kathleen drives herself to perform, but I'm concerned about her weight; she's beginning to look like a stick drawing when she takes off her practice sweats," the teacher said. "In this field we see a lot of girls who take things a bit too seriously and end up with major health problems."

At the teacher's repeated prompting, Kathleen's mother took her to see their pediatrician. Kathleen had hidden from her mother the fact that she hadn't menstruated in more than six months, just as she had covered up a dramatic weight loss by wrapping herself in baggy, oversized shirts, sweatpants, and leg-warmers.

"We call Kathleen's condition anorexia nervosa. It is a serious disorder and requires the attention of a specially qualified treatment team," the pediatrician noted. "I'm going to refer you to an eating disorders clinic where your whole family will get the help you need."

The doctor assured Kathleen's parents that the clinic had an excellent record in the treatment of eating disorders, but he warned that treatment can be difficult and it usually takes a long time. Relapses are common.

Who Develops Eating Disorders?

At least five million Americans suffer from various eating disorders: undereating, binge eating, or gorging and purging to prevent weight gain. The true number is difficult to judge, because

BEAUTY IS MORE THAN SKIN DEEP

> Help your children to feel comfortable with who they are. Encourage them to discover and develop their natural talents, no matter how modest, and to look beyond appearances in finding others to admire.

many people manage to hide their eating problems even from those closest to them. Once thought to be restricted to middle- and upper-income families, eating disorders are increasingly found at every social and economic level.

Eating disorders are most common in girls between ages 14 and 17, but are also seen in adolescent boys and young children. Overall, girls with eating disorders outnumber boys by about 10 to 1. Despite the increasing frequency of the problem, it's not yet possible to identify those who are likely to develop eating disorders. The roots of the problem appear to be complex. Outside influences play on internal factors in fostering eating disor-

ders. For example, magazines, movies, and television promote thinness as an ideal to aspire to. Most young people can deal with the message, but the one who develops an eating disorder is more susceptible and cannot keep it in perspective.

No age group is immune. Eating disorders in children under age 14 are described as "childhood onset." Some women secretly persist in eating disorders from their teens into their 20s, 30s, and beyond. Others develop bizarre eating behaviors in response to stress long after adolescence is over. Disordered eating is an occupational hazard among those whose jobs make unusual weight demands, such as high-fashion models, dancers, and professional athletes.

Jackie, at 18, was tall and slim and a rising star in track and field. A rigorous training schedule kept her muscles toned and allowed her to eat as much as she wanted. When a scout for a modeling agency tapped her at a regional track meet, Jackie's parents agreed to let her travel East with a view to launching a modeling career.

Jackie had always taken pride in looking her

RISKS FOR ADOLESCENT ATHLETES

High-school and college athletes are particularly susceptible to eating disorders. For example, coaches may encourage wrestlers to develop strength by training above their weight limits but competing at a lower weight, just under the limit. This means that a wrestler may be pressured to lose several pounds in just a few days before a competition. Adolescent athletes are often urged to follow unbalanced weight-loss regimens (for example, eating only bananas or oranges for days on end). Several college wrestlers have died when trying to make weight by going without food and water and working out while wearing special clothing to promote sweating. These practices are unsafe. Athletics coaches should be responsible for encouraging healthful eating and exercise. Parents who suspect that their young athletes are subjected to abusive practices should bring their concerns to the attention of school or college authorities.

If you answer YES to several of these questions, talk to your child and your pediatrician.

- Does your child skip family meals and prepare her own food instead?

- Is she following her own diet?

- Is she overly concerned with losing or gaining weight?

- Have you found laxatives that you did not give her?

- Does she hide food in her room?

- Does she spend long periods in the bathroom after eating?

- Has your plumbing repeatedly and inexplicably become plugged up?

- Does she have an unusual number of scratches or cuts over her knuckles?

- Has she lost a lot of weight in a short time?

- Does she look gaunt?

- Have her periods stopped?

- Does she toy with her food, without actually eating it?

- Has she developed downy hair on her face and arms?

- Does she wear loose, bulky clothing?

- Does she exercise for hours on end?

well-groomed best. But she was first puzzled, then angry, and finally disillusioned when executives at the agency evaluated her appearance. They told her she'd have to stop running, to prevent muscle development. They also told her to follow an extremely low-calorie diet to strip 15 pounds from her already slender body, and suggested she start smoking to help shed the weight and keep it off.

After talking it over with her parents, Jackie decided that a modeling career was not for her. She took the next flight home to begin her college applications and resume the sports in which she excelled.

Many young women who are attracted by promises of the wealth and glamour of a modeling career are not as clear-eyed as Jackie. In their efforts to achieve the perfect form for photographic modeling (far different from the average woman's shape), some adopt practices that are detrimental to health and can develop into eating disorders. Dancers and some athletes such as gymnasts are often susceptible to similar pressures.

The three principal eating disorders are: anorexia nervosa, or self-starvation; bulimia, or binge eating followed by purging through induced

Be on the lookout for diet fads, especially with adolescent girls. Some, such as high-protein, low-carbohydrate regimens, which are dangerously inadequate, have been around for decades and resurface periodically under new names. Over-the-counter diet aids, especially those with herbal ingredients such as ephedra or the related compound ephedrine are also widely used and dangerous. These compounds speed the heart rate and raise blood pressure; ephedra has been linked to several hundred deaths.

vomiting or laxative abuse to prevent weight gain; and bulimarexia, starvation alternating with gorging and induced purging. Irrespective of the specific behavior and diagnosis, those with eating disorders share a preoccupation with their weight and shape, have a severely erratic or inadequate food intake, and cannot regulate their eating.

Girls who start menstruating earlier than their peers tend to have more problems with body image and a somewhat higher risk of eating disorders. Offspring of parents with a history of eating disorders are also more vulnerable.

Anorexia Nervosa

Apart from drastic weight loss, the effects of anorexia include failure to menstruate and a growth of fine hair over the limbs and body. The body temperature drops and the skin feels oddly cool to the touch. Despite a woefully inadequate intake of calories, those with anorexia are often remarkably animated and energetic. They may exercise for hours on end to burn off the calories from something they've eaten. Many have trouble sleeping. Most are severely constipated because the intestinal muscles are weakened, the body's metabolism slows down, and the intake of food, fluid, and fiber is not enough to keep the bowel moving. Some anorexics drink large amounts of water before medical examinations, to try to hide weight loss.

Without treatment, a person with anorexia develops severe nutritional deficiencies and dehydration. In extreme cases (up to 5 out of every 100) the final result is death due to abnormal heart rhythm or other effects of starvation.

Like many girls with anorexia nervosa, Kathleen was a high achiever who pushed herself to perform. Also like many anorexics, Kathleen was preoccupied with food: cooking it, serving it to others, toying with it, and analyzing every last calorie and nutrient. The only thing she didn't do with food was eat normal amounts. When she ate at all, she tried to work off the calories with punishing exercise. Although on one level Kathleen persisted in the delusion that she was fat, on another she recognized that she looked abnormal, because she took pains to conceal her increasing emaciation under layers of bulky clothing. This had the further advantage, as she saw it, of promoting weight loss through perspiration.

If you suspect that your child is starving herself, seek professional help. Anorexia is a life-threatening condition, and one of its effects is to hinder the person's ability to make rational decisions concerning her own health. The only effective approach is a team effort providing nutrition counseling, medical care, and psychotherapy. Members of the treatment team involve the parents when appropriate. However, as with other aspects of eating, the main goal is to empower the affected person (here, the anorexic) to assume responsibility for her own nutrition.

A person under treatment for anorexia nervosa passes through three phases. In the first, the eating disorder itself is the focus of attention. Second, an improvement in dietary intake is offset by a shift in attitude; the anorexic becomes hostile and sullen. Finally, the anorexic begins to eat more normally and is more pleasant and cooperative. A successful transition from the second to the third phase indicates the best chance of long-term recovery; in other words, eating normally and maintaining an appropriate weight. About one third of anorexics have long-term problems coping with food and accepting a normal weight. The younger the child is when anorexia develops, the poorer the chances of recovery.

Bulimia Nervosa

Stacy, at age 14, was already a veteran of the diet wars. Her figure-conscious mother waged a continual battle, counting calories, serving commercial diet meals, and pinning her hopes on "miracle" diet supplements and formulas. In her mother's presence, Stacy dutifully nibbled on calorie-controlled portions and salads without dressing. Her weight stayed the same, however, and truth to tell, Stacy wasn't fat. She had simply inherited the stocky build of her father's side of the family.

What nobody else knew, however, was that at least once or twice a week, Stacy went on an eating binge. Her allowance easily covered a couple of quarts of ice cream and packages of chocolate chip cookies, a whole pizza with sausage and extra cheese, party-size bags of potato chips and cheese snacks, quarts of soda pop, sometimes an entire cheesecake from the frozen-foods section of the supermarket. Many or most of these and more went down at the same time, depending on how tense and upset she felt. The tension she felt beforehand was nothing, of course, compared with the shame she felt when the binge was over. But she found a way to fix that. As soon as the urge to binge began to wear off, Stacy would stick her fingers down her throat and bring it all up again. She felt bad for a while, because her stomach and throat hurt. "It's just my period,"

▷ **EATING DISORDER EMERGENCY**

If your child has an eating disorder and develops a rapid or irregular heartbeat, chest pain, or fainting, or if her weight loss continues, call your pediatrician at once. She may have a life-threatening complication.

Stacy replied when her mother once asked what was going on in the bathroom. She was always careful to throw out empty food packages away from her house.

Stacy was ashamed of the bingeing, but told herself it wasn't wrecking her calorie intake. After all, she got rid of most of the calories before her body could absorb them.

As Stacy approached college age, she wanted to be as slender as the more popular girls in her class. Reasoning that what worked for bingeing would work even better every day, Stacy began to finish off every dinner with her bathroom routine. She knew she needed a certain amount of food, so she kept her purging for the major meal of the day. Besides, the mornings were too rushed and school lunchtimes were difficult.

When a dental checkup revealed erosion of the

enamel on her rear teeth, the dentist called Stacy's mother. "I think you'd better talk to Stacy and call your pediatrician," he said. "Her teeth look as if they've been in an acid bath. This is the sort of problem we see in young people with eating disorders. They throw up so much that the stomach acid actually erodes the teeth."

After examining Stacy, her pediatrician recommended evaluation at a clinic that offered a team approach to the management of eating disorders.

For some bulimics, vomiting is a way to release built-up emotional tension in addition to ridding the body of calories. Many people practice vomiting even without gorging as a misguided method of weight control. Bulimics are skillful at hiding their disorder, and may binge and purge for years undiscovered. A telltale sign may be scratches on the knuckles or back of the hand, caused by the teeth when the bulimic pushes her fingers down her throat.

These conditions are difficult to diagnose because people with bulimia or bulimarexia are often of normal weight or, in the case of bulimia, even a little plump. In contrast to anorexics, bulimic girls usually do not lose their periods, because their weight and body fat rarely fall below critical levels. They can, however, have mood swings, swollen glands in the neck and face, stomach pain, and sore throats. The repeated vomiting creates an acid bath that burns the mucous membrane lining the esophagus and erodes the tooth enamel. Chronic heartburn and dental problems are among the consequences. In severe cases, a bulimic may hemorrhage from the esophagus and develop a dangerous imbalance of potassium and other salts, which can lead to disturbances in the heart rhythm. Once vomiting is established as a means of coping, bulimia can be difficult to treat. The person has to be willing to accept help. If you suspect bulimia in your child, talk to her and consult your pediatrician, who may provide a referral to an eating disorders clinic or recommend a psychotherapist experienced in treating adolescents with such problems.

Binge-Eating Disorder

Like bulimics, binge eaters repeatedly gorge on enormous quantities of food, sometimes equal to several days' worth of calories at once. Binges are typically followed by intense feelings of guilt and shame. Unlike bulimics, however, binge eaters do not purge themselves with vomiting or laxatives. As a result, they are usually (but not always) overweight. It's estimated that about 2 out of every 100 adolescents and adults are binge eaters. They seldom have outward physical symptoms other than weight gain, but they are at risk for problems associated with obesity, including high blood pressure, elevated blood cholesterol levels, gall bladder disease, and diabetes.

As with bulimia, binge eating can be difficult to diagnose, although it may emerge in the course of consultations for a weight problem. Sometimes, parents get their first clue that a young person is binge eating when food inexplicably disappears from the kitchen. If you are concerned about your child's weight or eating, talk to him or her and discuss it with your pediatrician.

Recovery

The team approach to treatment of eating disorders involves psychotherapy, medical intervention, and nutrition counseling. The treatment of anorexia nervosa is usually in two phases. During the recovery phase, medical problems are treated and eating is gradually reintroduced until weight returns to normal. In the maintenance phase, efforts are made to maintain normal eating patterns and prevent a relapse.

Because many anorexics have an aversion to food and cannot eat much at a time, calories are spread out through the day by way of snacks and mini-meals. A healthy goal weight is generally higher than the level that feels comfortable to an anorexic, so weight gain can be an uphill battle. Relapses are common.

Treatment for bulimia and binge eating involves teaching the young person to eat in response to hunger rather than to such inappropriate cues as loneliness or boredom. In contrast to anorexia nervosa, the goal is not weight gain if weight is within normal range or higher. Instead, the aim of treatment is to maintain weight while learning a new pattern of eating. Those who are overweight must learn how to eat and exercise normally in order to achieve and maintain a healthy weight.

With all eating disorders, the various ways in which family members express themselves, relate to one another, and handle stress can feed into the child's feelings of lack of control and make the situation worse. Treatment that involves the whole family can change the dynamics for the better, and help the person with the eating disorder.

ISSUES PARENTS RAISE ABOUT EATING DISORDERS

We've been advised to see a doctor because the school nurse thinks our daughter may have an eating disorder. Her weight is normal and she's very energetic, so how could this be?
Eating disorders sometimes remain undetected because the victims are of normal weight or even overweight. However, treatment is necessary to prevent serious effects on health (see p. 150). Talk to your pediatrician and follow any recommendations he or she may make for further consultations and treatment.

Do children with eating disorders start out as picky eaters?
Picky eaters may remain picky eaters (see p. 65), but they do not necessarily develop eating disorders. Despite the growing frequency of eating disorders, it's not yet possible to identify children at risk. Eating disorders are most common in girls between ages 14 and 17, but they are also seen in adolescent boys and younger children. In fact, they can occur at any age (see p. 146).

The high school wrestling coach told my son to eat nothing but apples for the next 4 days so he can make weight for a competition. Is this a safe way to lose weight?
This is a dangerous practice and it is banned by school and college athletics authorities. Keep your son on a balanced diet with plenty of fluids when he exercises, and report the coach's irresponsible advice to the high school. (Also see p. 146.)

CHAPTER 11

What Do I Do About Outside Influences?

When 7-year-old Greg demanded salt to shake over his meal, his mother refused. The food was well seasoned, she explained, and it isn't good for our bodies to eat too much salt.

"Dad always puts a lot of salt on his food, so is he going to get sick?" Greg countered.

Startled by the first-grader's awareness, Greg's father agreed that he often added salt from force of habit, even before tasting his food. Greg's parents stopped putting the salt shaker out on the table and Greg was pleased that his watchfulness might help Dad stay healthy.

You will soon find out—if you don't know it already—that your child's eating habits are affected by a lot more than your good advice. Friends, grandparents, childcare providers, and, last but certainly not least, television and magazine advertisements have a great influence over children's food likes and dislikes.

An Influential Role

As a parent, you have the first and possibly the most lasting influence on your child. That is true of many things, including food. You may not realize it, but every time you eat, you're setting an example for your child. He is likely to be influenced by what, how, where, when, and with whom you eat. By watching you, your child begins to form his own ideas of the "right" way to eat. This is especially true from birth through his preschool years, and you continue to have an impact even through the stormy teenage years—although that may be difficult to believe when you watch adolescents' behavior.

While your influence is great, you don't have to be a dictator. Rather, try to take a matter-of-fact approach. Simply keep your kitchen stocked with healthful foods and prepare appealing meals on a regular schedule. Let your child see that you eat healthful foods and moderate amounts. As a parent, you should control what foods are brought into the house, and you can be a healthy role model. But you cannot and should not watch over your child's shoulder. The older your children are, the less likely they are to respond positively to such supervision, and they may do exactly the opposite of what you've intended.

It's important to remember that as the parent, you are responsible for putting healthful meals on the table. It is your child's responsibility to eat them. Force-feeding is never the answer. Young children's appetites come and go with different stages of development—often even from day to day. Accept these changes, knowing that your child will probably make up for a lack of appetite today by eating heartily later in the week. If, however, lack of appetite becomes a chronic, long-term problem, talk it over with your child's pediatrician. In older children, especially girls, a chronic lack of appetite could be the sign of an eating disorder. (See Chapter 10.)

For younger children, avoid giving food as a reward or withholding it as a form of punishment. Bribery doesn't work. Threatening to withhold ice cream if your child doesn't eat her peas, or not allowing her to watch her favorite television show unless she cleans her plate, will only backfire. Such threats exaggerate the value of the "carrot" being dangled—in this case, ice cream or television. Moreover, a child who is pressured to eat may end up eating less than one who is allowed to choose what and how much to eat from what's offered.

For older children, unless what they're eating is actually harmful, avoid passing judgment. Doing so will only make matters worse. Your child's latest dietary dos and don'ts may be nothing more than a passing phase.

Lifestyle Logistics

When both parents work outside the home and older children are involved with outside activities, such as sports, dance, or scouting, every minute of family time counts. Much of that family time is likely to be mealtime. To make the most of it, don't let television take the place of talking to one another. Nor is a meal the time to read the newspaper or air grievances with other family members. Because family time is precious, try to make the time spent together at meals an opportunity for talking and listening rather than arguments and confrontations. A peaceful atmosphere increases the chance that your child or teenager will talk about his day. It also makes it more likely that young children will taste and accept new foods. By doing your best to create a welcoming atmosphere, you'll make mealtimes occasions the whole family looks forward to with pleasure.

Unfortunately, for many families family mealtime is more a memory than a reality. When the entire family is in a constant time crunch, with no time to sit down for family meals, nutrition suffers. Fast food and take-out become a habit, especially for evening meals. When both parents work outside the home, teenagers may be responsible for many of their own meals and those of younger siblings. Fast food offers an easy solution. But fast food doesn't have to mean bad food. There are lower-fat options at many fast food restaurants. With just a little planning, you can point your family in the direction of these

 WE DON'T NEED TO ADD SALT TO FOOD

Table salt is made up of sodium and chloride, two chemicals that are essential for health but only in very small amounts. Sodium and chloride occur naturally in many foods and it's not necessary to add them. A balanced diet based on the Food Guide Pyramid (p. 90) contains more than enough sodium to meet our daily requirement of 500 milligrams. Americans on average eat the equivalent of 1 to 3 teaspoons of salt a day, adding up to between 2,300 and 6,900 milligrams of sodium. One teaspoon a day is more than enough.

We add salt to food from force of habit or because we've learned to like a salty taste. Adding salt to food probably is not bad, except for those with high blood pressure who are extra-sensitive to sodium. Still, it's a good idea to train children to avoid unnecessary salt. One way is to keep the salt shaker off the dinner table. Taste food *before* you add salt and other seasonings.

▷ MAKING MORE HEALTHFUL CHOICES

INSTEAD OF	CHOOSE
∟ Pan-crust pepperoni pizza with extra cheese	Thin-crust vegetarian pizza with a sprinkling of cheese
∟ Cheeseburger with fries	Grilled chicken sandwich with baked potato
∟ Beef burrito with sour cream and cheese	Bean burrito with lettuce, tomato, and salsa
∟ Chicken nuggets with fries	Chicken fajita with salad and low-fat dressing

more healthful foods and still get them fed in the limited time available.

If family meals are rare during the workweek at your house, try to make at least one meal on the weekend—say Sunday dinner—a time when everyone is expected to take part. And do your best to set the example you wish you had time for during the week by serving a variety of healthful foods.

Childcare Providers

When Deborah Jackson went back to work three days a week, she was lucky to find a kind, active caregiver who looked after her two children with grandmotherly concern. The children looked forward to the caregiver's visits. They loved their daily reward of candy "for being good" and the potato chips and chocolate chip cookies she regularly served as after-school snacks.

When Deborah became aware of these snacks, she approached the problem as if speaking to her own mother. "The children are so happy, they feel they've practically got a new grandma. And I can go back to work with peace of mind.

"But we have our own way of doing things. I prefer to serve carrots and celery sticks or crackers and cheese for after-school snacks, and we save cookies for special treats. When it comes to being

good, a word of praise is enough; they don't need candy. It's fine for a treat once in a while, but I worry about their teeth if they have it every day."

Deborah backed up the discussion by writing daily instructions that always ended with a cheerful note of thanks. If her caregiver privately thought Deborah was a bit misguided, she kept it to herself and went along with Deborah's wishes.

Regardless of whether you're an at-home parent or work outside the home, chances are that at some point in your child's life you'll have to deal with outside influences on what your child eats. That holds true whether it's a live-in nanny, the teenager across the street, or a group-care worker who's looking after your child. How you handle different influences depends on who's doing the feeding. Your neighbor's teenage daughter will probably readily take instructions about what your child should and shouldn't eat. If she does not follow instructions well, she probably won't be getting too many more baby-sitting jobs.

A live-in nanny should also be willing to follow your wishes about feeding your child. But if your caregiver is older and has children of her own, or comes from another culture with different ideas about food, it could be more of a challenge to make sure your child gets the foods you want him to have. You and your caregiver may agree to disagree about what food is right, but be firm in letting her know how you would like your child's meals prepared. Be specific; the clearer your instructions, the less likely it is you'll have disagreements. If you work full-time, chances are your caregiver will feed more meals and snacks to your child than you do. So it's crucial to communicate for your child's good nutrition and your peace of mind.

What your child eats at a childcare center is less within your control. When selecting a care center, look into the food selections and how meals are served. If you're not satisfied with the food provided, speak with the director to find out if changes can be made or your child can brown-bag meals and snacks. If you're able to pack your child's meals and snacks for the day (some places require it, but others don't allow it), include whole-grain breads, cereals, or crackers; a source of protein, such as lean meat, egg, or peanut butter; and fruits and vegetables.

Family Food Feuds

You work hard at putting food on the table. You read labels, select foods of good quality, and try out new, healthful recipes. Don't let critical comments from visiting family members throw you off balance. Your father may grumble that there's not enough meat on the table, or your mother may insist that your 5-year-old needs whole-fat milk to stay healthy. Remember that they mean well. However, as the parent in charge of this household, you control what's put on the table.

If it's your mother or mother-in-law who's offering feeding advice, the situation may have to be handled with special finesse. After all, these women come with experience and memories of rearing and feeding their own children. As they see it, their offspring turned out all right, so what's wrong with the way they did things? Don't give them a lecture on how times have changed, or why your meals are more nutritious and healthful than theirs were. You'll invite a confrontation, and power struggles over food only create an uncomfortable mood at the dinner table. Feelings may be hurt unless suggestions are made tactfully. Instead of "Don't force any more food on Tim," it may be more helpful to say, "We've learned that Tim likes to decide for himself how much to eat," or rather than, "Don't overload Bobby's plate," try "Bobby has an easier time eating if you only offer one or two foods at a time." Or try recruiting your mother's or mother-in-law's help. "Mom, I need a hand. Could you feed the baby while I finish getting the dinner?" If your dad wants more meat on the table, budget your family's fat intake to allow a roast or steak dinner when he visits.

What to do about comments from other family members? Thank them for their suggestions, chalk them up to differences of opinion, and let it go. You may never truly see eye to eye, but you all have the same goal: to do the best for your children and see them grow up healthy and strong.

Peer Pressure

On weeknights, 3-year-old Stephanie ate earlier than her parents, because her father didn't get home from work until close to her bedtime. Stephanie's mother planned meals carefully but sometimes allowed the preschooler a choice for supper. Stephanie set a personal record for consistency by asking for spaghetti with tomato-vegetable sauce every night for two weeks in a row (except on the weekend, when she ate dinner with her parents). On the 15th evening, Stephanie threw a tantrum when she saw her mother reach for the pasta box. "No spaghetti!" she shrieked. "I hate bad worms!"

Stephanie's mother was relieved that the

▷ LUNCH-BOX ALTERNATIVES FOR GOOD NUTRITION

- Whole-wheat bread is out? Try a high-fiber white bread. There are a few brands on the market now.

- They want bologna? Try a low-fat turkey bologna instead of beef.

- The apple is now a thing of the past? Try applesauce or a different fruit.

- Chips are a must? Replace greasy, salty potato chips with low-fat baked tortilla chips, or try a reduced-fat, low-salt brand of potato or vegetable chips.

spaghetti craze was over. While it made meals easy, it certainly was boring. When Stephanie calmed down, however, she revealed that her best friend at childcare had let her in on a big secret: Spaghetti with red sauce was made with worms and blood, and no 3-year-old in her right mind should eat it.

Stephanie's parents bought pasta in different shapes and experimented with different sauces until the great worm scare was forgotten.

As a parent, you should brace yourself for unexpected influences to affect your children as early as age 2 1/2. By this time, most children are talking and beginning to socialize with siblings and neighbors, in play groups, or with others in preschool or childcare. Food likes and dislikes among toddlers and school-age children can vary from day to day. While a food may have been your child's favorite for weeks, even months, don't be surprised if it's suddenly blacklisted. This may simply be a toddler's fickle tastes or the result of another child telling her that it's disgusting.

When he reaches school age, your child's focus will shift away from the home toward friends, teachers, and outside activities. The sphere of influences affecting him will grow wider, while what you do will seem somewhat less important.

You may begin to see the effects of peer pressure

early on, when your first-grader decides she no longer wants whole-wheat bread for her sandwiches, because her best friend always has white bread. Other children will ask what's in her lunch box and tell her what they think of it. There are ways to make the experience easier on your child while still giving her the good nutrition you want her to have.

In early adolescence and later, your child's friends are likely to have a growing influence on what, when, and how he eats. As with many other aspects of life, from dress to language, adolescents are likely to make food choices with little more in mind than what their friends think. Because adolescents are self-conscious about their changing bodies and may not be completely comfortable with the changes taking place, concern with size and shape can easily cross over into obsession. That makes adolescence a high-risk time for eating disorders such as anorexia nervosa and bulimia. But because our society as a whole values thinness, while obesity is often viewed as a character defect rather than a disorder, it is sometimes tough to tell when a teenager's preoccupation has crossed the line. (Also see Chapter 10.) While girls' concerns most often center on thinness, boys pay more attention to muscle develop-

Low-fat yogurt	Prepackaged, precut vegetables with low-fat dips
Fresh fruit	Low-fat pudding
High-fiber, unsweetened cereals	1percent fat or skim milk
Nuts	Low-fat cottage cheese
Low-fat microwave popcorn	Dried fruit
Reduced-fat cheese	Rice cakes
Peanut butter	Whole-grain crackers
Bagels	Whole-wheat bread
Low-fat lunch meats, cold cuts	Pita bread
Pretzels	Reduced-fat mayonnaise and/or fat-free dressings
Tofu	Baked tortilla chips
Bean dip, chickpea spread (hummus), eggplant dip	Microwaveable, low-fat entrées (enchiladas, burritos, pasta with chunky tomato and vegetable sauce)
Low-fat granola bars	Salsa

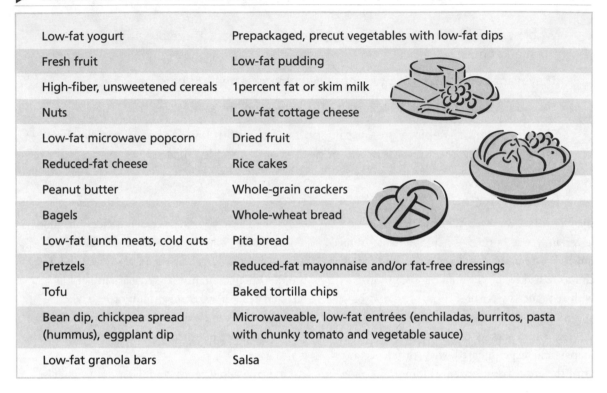

ment. High-priced products such as protein powders and amino acid supplements promise Arnold Schwarzenegger–like bodies but deliver little more than unnecessary protein.

While your teenager may amaze you at the sheer quantities of food he can eat in one sitting, try not to become a food monitor. If your teenager is normally active, chances are he'll naturally regulate his own intake. Because weight is such a pressing concern for adolescent girls, parental watchfulness together with warnings of eating too much could have the opposite effect to what you intend. Your teenager may eat more than normal just to prove she is in control.

As your adolescent matures and learns more about food and nutrition from other sources, it's likely he'll begin to develop his own opinions. He may begin to experiment with different food styles, such as vegetarianism. Try not to react negatively. Rather, listen to the reasons behind his decision and try to be supportive. Learn as much as you can about this new eating style, so you can help your teenager use it to achieve a nutritionally balanced diet. (Also read about alternative diets and supplements in Chapter 14.) Now is a good time to shift responsibility for some shopping and food preparation on to your child, especially if his new eating style is different from that of the rest of the family. However, if the new way of eating seems unhealthy, then it is your responsibility to explain why it's not a good idea. Round up some reading material that supports what you're saying if your teenager is unwilling to accept your opinions about food fads or even junk foods. It becomes even more important to provide healthful choices when the family eats together because you have a diminishing influence on what your adolescent eats outside the home. If your teenager is always on the run, coming in to eat at odd hours long after the table has been cleared, keep the kitchen stocked with nutritious, easy-to-fix foods and snacks that you know he or she will eat. If you lay a good foundation at home, chances are your teenager will do just fine, in spite of temptations and distractions.

Limit the Influence of TV

Like it or not, television has a major impact on most of our lives. The Stevens family had a single television set, and when it broke, they never got around to having it fixed. For a year and a half, they lived without television and didn't miss it. Naomi Stevens's mother stayed with the family for a few months between the time her house was sold and her new condominium was ready. She brought her TV with her.

"All of a sudden, I found myself alone in the kitchen making dinner every night," Naomi said. "Before, everyone used to help with setting the table and cooking. After dinner, we would sit around the table and talk for a while.

"When that TV came into the house, the kids raced into the den and argued over what show they would watch. I was glad when Mom's condo was finally ready. We could get back to being a family that talked again."

After the family, television is probably the most important influence on child development and behavior in our society. That behavior includes your child's eating habits. Children in the United States view an average of 3 to 4 hours of television a day. By the time the average

teenager graduates from high school, he or she has spent more time watching television than in the classroom. Not surprisingly, research has shown that young people who watch a lot of television are less physically fit, because TV watching takes time away from play and other physical activity. In many cases, television exerts a subtle and destructive influence on the family's eating habits and communication around the table.

Set firm limits on TV viewing and the time spent on computer and video games (which must be nonviolent). Join your children outdoors and get the whole family moving. For young children, arrange playdates so they have something to occupy their time besides sitting in front of the

▷ TELEVISION TACTICS

The cardinal rule at mealtime is: "Turn off the television." As your children grow, meals together become rare and precious opportunities for family interaction. Make the most of them by eliminating as many distractions as possible. Television is probably the worst offender.

television or computer. For older children, encourage extracurricular activities such as tennis, soccer, football, gymnastics, volleyball, swimming, in-line skating, and dance. When possible, make physical activity a family affair by going for walks or bike rides together.

On television, your child sees one sales pitch after another designed to convince consumers they want things they don't need. The average child sees more than 20,000 commercials each year; that's more than 60 a day. A large number of

In 1990, Congress passed the Children's Television Act to make sure that TV stations pay attention to the needs of child viewers. Under this law, stations must air educational and informational shows for children, and limit the amount of advertising during those shows to 12 minutes per hour on weekdays and $10^1/2$ minutes per hour on weekends. If this law is to be effective, consumers have to act as watchdogs. Keep tabs on TV stations in your area and report any violation to the Federal Communications Commission. Send a written complaint to the Chief, Mass Media Bureau, FCC, 1919 M Street N.W., Washington, D.C. 20554.

them are food commercials, strategically placed during children's TV programs, and mostly for high-calorie and/or high-fat foods such as candy, snacks, and presweetened cereals. In fact, more than 40 percent of all commercials that children see are for sugared cereals, candy, fatty foods, and toys. Commercials for meat, milk products, bread, and juice, on the other hand, make up only about 4 percent of the food ads shown during children's programming, and ads for fruits and vegetables are virtually nonexistent.

It stands to reason, then, that TV would play a role in childhood obesity. Research bears that out. Indeed, the risk of being overweight is more than $4^1/2$ times greater for children who watch more than 5 hours of television a day compared with children who watch no more than 2 hours a day.

Don't expect your child to be able to resist ads for candy and snack foods without your help. When your child asks for a product he saw advertised on TV, explain how TV makes him want things he does not need—even things that could be harmful. Be specific: Point out the commercials you're talking about. When a commercial plugging a children's cereal comes on, explain why advertisers chose to buy time during his favorite show. Explain that the advertisers want

people to buy cereal and are not necessarily concerned with his well-being. Children often do not understand the purpose of commercials until it is spelled out for them. Your child may nag, whine, cry, and try to cajole you into buying unhealthful foods, but be firm and ignore it as well as you can. Once you begin negotiating over junk food, you've already lost the battle.

Here are some tips for avoiding ads that sell nutritionally poor products to your children:

- Choose public television over commercial TV whenever possible.
- Tape programs for your children for watching at a later time, and edit out or fast-forward through the commercials.

▷ HOW MUCH TV IS ENOUGH?

The average child watches 3 to 4 hours of television a day, but 1 to 2 hours a day of good quality TV programming and video or computer games combined is the maximum recommended by the American Academy of Pediatrics.

- Build up a family library of child-friendly favorite videos.

Children are particular targets for commercials advertising fast-food restaurants. These chains attract children with promotional tie-ins for toys. The playgrounds at some locations are hard to resist. Some pediatricians have observed, only half-jokingly, that children's ability to recognize chain restaurant logos has become something of a developmental milestone.

It's true that most items at fast-food restaurants are relatively low in valuable nutrients such as vitamin C, iron, and vitamin A and high in saturated fat, cholesterol, and sodium. However, some menus offer more nutritious, low-fat options, such as grilled chicken sandwiches, reduced-fat milk, and salads. If your child never swerves from his choice of a saturated-fat-heavy burger and fries, cut down on trips to fast-food outlets. The clogging of arteries from atherosclerosis, which sets the stage for heart disease, begins in childhood and is influenced by the amount of fat in the diet. Keep trips to fast-food restaurants as treats, rather than as routine meals. If your family's usual diet is well balanced and low in fat, an occasional burger and fries isn't going to be harmful. But frequent consumption of high-fat foods, like hot dogs, burgers, and fries, is unhealthy for adults and children alike.

In adolescence, your child's friends are likely to have the strongest influence over her choices. Here, too, television is important, and fast food outlets also play a major role in the lives of teenagers. It's not clear whether that is due to the influence of television, friends, or both. But because fast-food restaurants offer affordable fare and a place to sit, they often serve as gathering spots.

To diminish the impact television has on your child, regardless of his age, the best thing you can do, as a parent, is to set limits on television viewing. First, be aware of how many hours of TV your child is in the habit of watching. Limit viewing time to 1 to 2 hours per day. Finally, keep the television under your control. That means no TV sets in the children's rooms. Be firm. If necessary, install "lock out" devices, which prevent young

▶ THE UNREAL WORLD OF TELEVISION COMMERCIALS

In television commercials, sports figures, supermodels, rock stars, and movie stars push everything from potato chips and fast food to soft drinks and dietary supplements. Slick ads imply that if you drink this soda, eat this food, or take this supplement you will be as confident, beautiful, slim, and fun-loving as the beautiful people in the ads. Because adolescence is a time of intense approval-seeking behavior, teenagers are especially vulnerable to the unspoken promises of self-improvement and acceptance in such ads. While most food ads are appealing, few promote overall healthful eating. In fact, some blatantly encourage overeating. Yet, paradoxically, the overwhelming majority of people in both television ads and shows are athletically built and uncommonly slim. Explain to your children that if the actors frequently snacked on the products they promoted, they wouldn't stay slim for long.

people from tuning in to selected channels, such as certain movie channels or adult programming.

Help your child become physically active. Television watching is synonymous with inactivity. And snacking while watching TV sets the stage for unwanted weight gain. The best approach is to limit TV viewing from your children's very earliest years, so they don't become dependent on television and video for entertainment and stimulation. If your child is used to watching more than a couple of hours of TV a day, or playing computer games or "surfing the net," it may take some effort to get him interested in other activities. Don't be surprised if your child rebels and even goes through a sort of "withdrawal" when you cut back on his TV time. And remember, your children look to you for example. It might be a good idea to take a critical look at your own television-viewing habits before you try to revamp those of your children.

ISSUES PARENTS OFTEN RAISE ABOUT OUTSIDE INFLUENCES

My toddler will be starting at a group childcare center soon, when I go back to work. I'm worried that she won't get healthful meals, the way she does at home.
Look into the food selections and how meals are served. If the center allows you to pack your child's meals and snacks for the day, include whole-grain breads, cereals, and crackers; a source of protein such as meat, fish, or low-fat cheese; and fruits and vegetables. (Also see p. 156.)

Both of us work full-time, so our teenager often has to get dinner for himself and his younger sister. We often let him order out for fast food. My kids seem to be growing okay, so is fast food as bad as some people say?

Fast food doesn't have to mean bad food. There are lots of lower-fat options, such as thin-crust vegetarian pizza with just a sprinkling of cheese, or chicken fajitas with salad and low-fat dressing. Stock your freezer with low-fat, microwaveable entrées. And if family mealtime is a rarity during the week, try to make at least one weekend meal a family dinner when everyone takes part. (Also see pp. 155 and 159.)

My first-grader refuses to take whole-wheat bread in her lunch box because her best friend always has white bread.
Lunch-box contents are inevitably examined and criticized. You can make it easier on your child while still giving her good nutrition. Make sandwiches with

Of course, television isn't the only arm of the media that reaches out to teenagers. Magazines aimed at adolescent readers offer nutrition information and advice, together with articles about dieting, alongside food advertising. While some columns and articles are responsible and accurate, others reinforce an adolescent's least healthy inclinations. Perhaps most disturbing are the images of overly thin models pushing products ranging from make-up and clothes to the latest dating advice. While you can't monitor all your adolescent's reading material, be aware that she may be turning to magazines as her main source of information about diet and health, and thus absorbing an unrealistic image of what the "ideal" body should be. Whether your teenager's goal is an ultra-slender figure, or the ultimate performance in her chosen sport, help her to be comfortable with herself and her body type through sound information and balanced nutrition.

high-fiber white bread. If she must have bologna, buy low-fat turkey bologna. Pack flavored applesauce if she won't take an apple. If she must have chips, replace greasy, salty potato chips with baked tortilla chips or reduced-fat, low-salt potato or vegetable chips. (For more tips, see p. 157.)

I try to keep my family on a healthy, low-fat diet, but when our folks visit, I hear nothing but criticism: "There's not enough meat here to feed a cat!" "These green vegetables are still half-raw." "I always gave you whole milk and you turned out all right."
Don't let family members' comments throw you off balance. They mean well, but this is your family now and you're in charge of what goes on the table. Avoid confrontation; it will only lead to an uncomfortable mood at the dinner table. Listen to their opinions and then enlist their help, where possible, in dealing with immediate, manageable needs such as playing with the baby or preparing vegetables. (For other, tips see p. 156)

My teenager has just announced she's going vegetarian. What'll I do?
A properly planned vegetarian diet is healthful and well balanced, and it can easily fit with regular family meals. Listen to the reasons behind your teenager's decision. Learn as much as you can so you can help her achieve a nutritionally balanced diet. Round up some reading material to help her plan meals. (Also see p. 158 and Chapter 14.)

Can I Cut My Child's Risk Of...?

In the course of a well-child visit for 5-year-old Sara, her mother mentioned that Sara's grandmother, 54 years old, had recently been hospitalized for a heart attack. Because of that, Sara's father had had his cholesterol level checked and it turned out to be high, about 260 mg/dl. He was now receiving treatment to lower his cholesterol and, with it, his risk of heart disease.

Routine cholesterol testing for all young children is not considered necessary. However, given the information about Sara's family, their pediatrician advised a blood test. Sara's results showed no sign of the high blood cholesterol that sometimes runs in families and can appear at a young age. Their pediatrician suggested that Sara's mother base family meal planning on the Food Guide Pyramid (see p. 90) and American Heart Association (AHA) recommendations for a carbohydrate-based diet. These guides advise no more than 30 percent of daily calories in the form of fat, with saturated fat making up no more than one third of total fats. He also suggested that Sara's parents strictly limit her television-viewing time and make time available for active play. When she was older, there'd be time for more structured exercise. Finally, although

Heredity is clearly an important risk factor for conditions such as heart disease, cancer, and diabetes. However, researchers are steadily amassing evidence that underscores the influence of diet on the development of diseases. Most research into the diet-health connection has been done in adults, but experts agree that healthy eating habits from an early age can lower the risk of developing several often deadly diseases later on. A diet designed to lower the risk of heart disease, cancer, and diabetes is one that benefits the whole family, adults and children alike.

Sara's cholesterol was normal, her pediatrician recommended periodic blood tests to catch any change early and provide for corrective steps.

Heart Disease

Heart disease is the number one killer of both men and women in the United States and most industrialized countries. The chief risk factors are smoking, high blood pressure, diabetes, a high blood level of cholesterol, physical inactivity, and overweight. If members of your family have had heart disease at an early age, your child, too, may be at risk for early-onset heart disease.

American children and adolescents, on average, eat more saturated fat and have higher blood cholesterol levels than young people their age in most other developed countries. The rate of heart disease tends to keep pace with cholesterol levels. One study found early signs of hardening of the arteries (atherosclerosis) in 7 percent of children between ages 10 and 15, and the rate was twice as high between ages 15 and 20. According to the AHA, a heart-healthy diet from an early age lowers cholesterol and, if followed through adolescence and beyond, should reduce the risk of coronary artery disease in adulthood.

▷ CHOLESTEROL TESTING FOR ADOPTED CHILDREN

Complete biological family medical histories are not usually available to adopted children and their parents, even for those adopted in open proceedings. To prevent the development of diseases linked to high blood cholesterol levels, adopted children should be screened periodically for blood lipid levels throughout childhood.

TESTING BLOOD CHOLESTEROL LEVELS. The American Academy of Pediatrics recommends cholesterol testing for two groups of children:

- Those whose parents or grandparents have had heart attacks or have been diagnosed with blocked arteries or disease affecting the blood vessels, such as stroke, before age 55.
- Those whose parents have blood cholesterol of 240 mg/dl or higher.

A child may have high cholesterol due to obesity, diabetes, liver disease, kidney disease, or an underactive thyroid. If an initial test shows high cholesterol, your pediatrician will check your child's blood again 2 weeks later to confirm the results. If it is still high, the doctor will also determine if your child has an underlying condition.

▷ CHOLESTEROL LEVELS IN CHILDREN AND ADOLESCENTS

Classification	Total Cholesterol*	Low-Density Lipoprotein (LDL)*
Acceptable	<170	<110
Borderline	170–199	110–129
High	>200	>130
*milligrams per 100 milliliters of blood		

DIET TO LOWER BLOOD CHOLESTEROL LEVELS. If a second blood test confirms that your child's blood cholesterol is high, a change in diet is the first approach to reducing it. Your pediatrician will probably recommend the AHA Step I Diet for a child over age 2 (see chart on following page). If you would like further guidance in planning a heart-healthy diet for your child (and most parents are glad to have some guidance), ask your pediatrician to refer you to a registered dietitian who specializes in children and families. Before you meet with the dietitian, you will probably be asked to keep a record of everything your child eats over the course of 3 to 7 days, to provide an idea of his eating patterns as well as his likes and dislikes.

Despite efforts to educate parents and children about healthy eating, and surveys showing that children and adolescents are eating less fat than they did 25 years ago, Americans of all ages are getting fatter (also see Chapter 8). Because overweight is one of the major risk factors for heart disease, maintenance of a healthy weight is crucial to reducing your child's risk of developing atherosclerosis and heart disease. (For more information on obesity and weight maintenance, see Chapter 8.) The AHA Diets for children are designed to reduce the intake of fat and cholesterol while helping to control weight and provide for growth.

If the cholesterol level has not dropped as much as your pediatrician would like after 3 months on the Step I Diet, you may be advised to follow the Step II Diet, which further cuts down on dietary fat and cholesterol. However, you should not try to reduce your child's fat or calorie intake without your pedia-

AMERICAN HEART ASSOCIATION STEP I AND STEP II DIETS

Nutrient	Step I Diet	Step II Diet
Total fat	Average of no more than 30% of total calories	Same as Step I
Saturated fat	Less than 10% of total calories	Less than 7% of total calories
Polyunsaturated fat	Up to 10% of total calories	Same as Step I
Monounsaturated fat	Remaining dietary fat calories	Same as Step I
Cholesterol	Less than 300 mg/day	Less than 200 mg/day
Carbohydrates	About 55% of total calories	Same as Step I
Protein	About 15% of total calories	Same as Step I
Calories	To promote growth and development	Same as Step I

trician's advice. Cutting back too much could adversely affect the number one childhood goal, which is normal growth and development. In particular, fat and cholesterol should not be restricted in children younger than 2. They need the calories from fat during this period of rapid development, when nutritional requirements are intense and restrictions could be harmful. The period beginning with the second birthday is a time of transition when you should decrease the fat and cholesterol content of your child's diet to the recommended levels. Thus, after age 2, he should be drinking skim or low-fat milk and getting no more than 30 percent of daily calories from fats, with one third or less of fat calories from saturated fats (see Chapters 6 and 13).

In addition to these guidelines, the National Cholesterol Education Program Expert Panel on Blood Cholesterol Levels in Children recommends that children eat a wide variety of foods, with enough calories to support normal growth and reach or maintain a healthy body weight. **FIBER AND CHOLESTEROL.** Not only is fiber impor-

tant to keep the digestive tract functioning smoothly, but it also helps regulate blood cholesterol. Diets rich in soluble fiber—the kind found in grains (especially oats), legumes and other vegetables, and fruits—have been shown to lower cholesterol levels in adults. Studies have not been performed to see whether these foods lower cholesterol in children. However, in all likelihood, fiber is equally beneficial at every age.

The AAP recommends that children consume fiber equal to $^1/_2$ gram per kilogram (2.2 pounds) of body weight per day, but not more than 35 grams. Pediatricians suggest a simpler way to calculate fiber: your child's age plus 5. Thus, for a 7-year-old, daily intake should be no less than 7 + 5 = 12 grams, up to a maximum of 35 grams.

You probably don't have to calculate your child's fiber intake in grams, because there should be plenty of fiber in a normal diet that includes at least five daily servings of vegetables and fruits, in addition to breads and cereals. However, if your child is constipated, or if she isn't getting five a day, try to increase her fiber intake. Avoid refined

Oils from plants such as rapeseed, or canola, flaxseed, and walnuts are good sources of linolenic acid, a fatty acid that our bodies convert to protective omega-3 fatty acids.

white flour and serve whole-grain breads, crackers, pasta, and cereals instead. Offer fruit or carrot sticks, celery, and other vegetables for snacks.

ONE FISH...TWO FISH... Adults who eat fish several times a week have a lower risk of heart disease than those who don't. The protective effect has been traced to omega-3 fatty acids, a special kind of fat found in fish.

Researchers haven't yet looked for evidence of comparable protection in children, but it's a good idea to make fish a regular part of your child's diet. Fatty fish like salmon, mackerel, and bluefish are especially rich sources of omega-3 fatty acids. When preparing fish, choose low-fat cooking methods such as broiling and steaming; deep-frying in batter only adds unnecessary fat and calories.

CHOLESTEROL-LOWERING MEDICATIONS. Pediatricians consider using cholesterol-lowering medications only when children age 10 years or older still have high cholesterol after 6 months to 1 year of dietary measures or have a family history of heart disease, or if the child is overweight or has an additional risk factor such as diabetes. The only medications the American Academy of Pediatrics currently approves for children are colestipol and cholestyramine. These compounds, known as bile acid binders, attach to molecules of bile acids, which help digest fats. Bile acids are made from cholesterol, and bile acids when bound to these

drugs pass out in the stool. Pediatricians prescribe these medications only after trying other methods, however, because of a small risk that they could interfere with growth.

PHYSICAL ACTIVITY. Surveys show that fewer than 25 percent of children in grades 4 through 12 get 30 minutes of physical activity every day, even though experts urge no less than 30 minutes of physical activity on most days of the week. Not only is exercise essential in maintaining a healthy weight, but aerobic activities such as soccer, basketball, track, skating, and jumping rope also strengthen the heart and lungs. To keep your child fit, make physical activity a family affair. Regulate TV time, and arrange for children to play outside. Go for family walks, hikes, and bicycle rides. Gather neighborhood young people for running bases, basketball games, or touch football. Regular exercise is just as important as a healthy diet in preventing heart disease.

Diabetes

People with diabetes are diagnosed according to whether they require insulin treatment (Type I), or can manage their condition with diet, exercise, and oral medications to control blood glucose levels (Type II). Type I diabetics do not produce insulin, a hormone made in the pancreas, which helps convert sugar into energy. Type II diabetics produce insulin but are resistant to its effects. Children most often develop Type I diabetes, which carries over into adulthood; adults are more likely to develop Type II, although many eventually require daily insulin injections.

Environmental factors such as viral infections, toxins, and emotional stress may trigger a child's genetic predisposition to Type I diabetes. It is called an "autoimmune" disease, in which the body mistakes its own tissue as unfamiliar. When

Children whose parents smoke are forced to breathe air fouled by poisons such as carbon monoxide, ammonia, nicotine, and hydrogen cyanide, as well as many cancer-causing compounds. The sidestream smoke that curls into the air from cigarettes carries even higher levels of toxins than the mainstream smoke that cigarette users inhale. Children of smokers suffer many more respiratory infections, asthma, and sudden infant deaths (SIDS) than children of nonsmokers. They are twice as likely to develop lung cancer in adult life as children of nonsmokers. Nonsmoking adults who spend years breathing the smoke from their partners' cigarettes have an increased risk of dying from heart disease due to an inadequate supply of oxygen to the heart. Long-term exposure to secondhand smoke also may put children at risk for heart disease in adulthood. The best thing you can do for your child's health is not to smoke, and not to allow smoking in your home. If you smoke, until you can stop, never smoke in the car, inside your home, or anywhere near your children.

that happens, the immune system turns on the pancreas as if it were a foreign invader and interferes with its ability to produce insulin. Those with Type I diabetes often have family histories of other autoimmune conditions, such as thyroid disorders or rheumatoid arthritis. Some researchers suggest that early exposure to cow's milk protein may, in some children, trigger destruction of the insulin-producing cells in the pancreas. Though this theory is unproved, the American Academy of Pediatrics recommends that parents avoid giving cow's milk for the first year to reduce the risk of Type I diabetes in children. Breastfeeding for at least the first year may protect against diabetes, in addition to its many other benefits.

Though Type II diabetes is more common in those over age 20, the incidence among youth is on the rise as children are getting heavier. Family history plays a role, but being overweight is probably the strongest risk factor of all. Reduce your child's risk of Type II diabetes by helping him maintain a healthy weight with a well-balanced diet and regular exercise. The healthy habits that you instill in childhood can help keep risk low in the adult years.

Cancer

As with heart disease, diet throughout life appears to influence the risk of various cancers. Interest in

 SYMPTOMS OF DIABETES

If your child has these symptoms, call your pediatrician at once:

- Weight loss
- Excessive thirst
- Frequent urination
- Dehydration with dry lips, sunken eyes, no tears when crying

A balanced diet, with plenty of calcium and vitamin D to increase calcium absorption, should provide all the nutrients necessary to build strong teeth and keep gums and mouth tissues healthy. Young people can get adequate calcium from three or four daily servings of dairy foods, as well as from many other sources: calcium-processed tofu, calcium-fortified orange juice, and green vegetables such as broccoli.

In areas where the natural fluoride content of the water is low and water supplies are not fluoridated, pediatricians and dentists may advise fluoride supplements (also see p. 35), or fluoride toothpaste or treatments to strengthen children's tooth enamel against decay.

All sugars promote the growth of mouth bacteria that produce acid and cause tooth decay. Unrefined sugars such as honey, maple syrup, and molasses are just as damaging as refined white sugar in this respect. The worst offenders are the sugars in sticky foods that cling to the teeth, such as dried fruit leathers and candies. Sodas and sweetened juice drinks leave the teeth awash in sugar. Cereals and other starchy foods, such as popcorn, leave a residue that bacteria rapidly convert to sugar.

However, while fructose, the sugar in fruits, can promote tooth decay, eating fruit also stimulates the flow of saliva, which helps to wash such naturally occurring sugars out of the mouth. The fats in walnuts and certain proteins and fats in Cheddar cheese appear to neutralize bacterial acids and may help to counteract their destructive effect. Tannins in tea and chocolate, among other foods, also seem to protect against cavities. Sweets are likely to be less harmful if eaten as part of a meal. Encourage youngsters to floss and brush after meals. When brushing is impossible (such as when out on a hike or in school), they should try to end a meal by drinking plain water or chewing on a firm, fibrous snack such as a carrot or celery stick to help remove food scraps and stimulate saliva flow.

fat as a cancer trigger began when researchers found that people in countries where the intake of fat—especially saturated fat—was high also had high rates of cancers of the breast, colon, prostate, ovary, and endometrium. More recent studies have found only weak connections between fat intake and breast cancer, but research continues to suggest a possible link between frequent consumption of red and processed meat and an increased risk for colon cancer. While there is some confusion about which cancers can be linked specifically to fat consumption, there's no doubt that a low-fat diet is associated with a lower overall risk for many diseases, including most types of cancer.

GRILLED AND BARBECUED FOODS. Chemicals that cause cancer can form during any cooking process. Some are even produced in the body during digestion. Scientists caution that a substance may have cancer-causing potential if it changes the DNA of bacteria cultured in the laboratory. High-heat methods of cooking meat, such as broiling, frying, and barbecuing, produce concentrations of DNA-altering chemicals that are about 50 times greater than those in baked and boiled meats. Hydrocarbons, including benzene, form when meat is broiled, and cancer-causing nitrosamines are produced both during cooking and in the digestive tract when processed meats containing nitrite, such as bacon, are eaten.

There's no call for undue alarm, however. As with all foods, moderation and balance are the key. It's a good idea to steam, bake, and braise most of the time, but there's no harm in grilling or barbecuing occasionally. Besides, you can take steps to reduce exposure to potentially harmful compounds.

Do all grilling and barbecuing in a well-ventilated area, to reduce exposure to carcinogens in smoke. Use a drip-pan with a spatter-proof shield to prevent fat from forming smoke. Reduce high-heat cooking time: Partially bake or parboil foods, then finish off with just a few minutes on the grill to add flavor.

Vitamins C and E block the chemical process that forms nitrosamines in the digestive tract. Phytates in wheat bran bind with nitrite and prevent nitrosamine formation. Bioflavonoids—pigments found in many fruits and vegetables—and other naturally occurring compounds known as phytochemicals are believed to block the action of many cancer-causing substances. So, when you have a barbecue, round out the meal with vegetables and fruits, as well as whole-grain breads and salads for bran, vitamins, and other natural cancer fighters.

Balance Is Best

There can be little doubt that childhood diets have an impact on the risk of disease in adulthood. Most evidence of factors that trigger disease is evaluated in statistical terms, as trends in vast numbers of people rather than as changes in individuals. However, evidence points toward a protective effect from a diet rich in grains, vegetables, and fruits, and with low levels of fats, particularly saturated fat. Serve at least one green and one yellow or red vegetable, plus a starchy vegetable or whole grain, every dinnertime and follow a "just-one-bite" policy. That is, even if your child claims not to like vegetables, ask that he try at least one bite of those on the plate. Serve fruits routinely for dessert, either alone or with cheese or yogurt. A habit of never eating fewer than five servings of fruits and vegetables a day may help reduce your child's risk of developing heart disease, cancer, diabetes, and other serious ailments later in life.

Should children have cholesterol checks just as adults do?

Pediatricians do not consider routine cholesterol testing to be necessary for all young children. However, if you have a family history of heart disease or your child is adopted, ask your pediatrician when cholesterol testing should be performed. (See p. 166.)

Is fiber all it's cracked up to be?

Not only is fiber important to keep the digestive tract functioning smoothly, but it also helps regulate blood cholesterol. Diets rich in soluble fiber—the kind found in grains (especially oats), legumes and other vegetables, and fruits—have been shown to lower cholesterol levels in adults. Studies have not been performed to see whether these foods lower cholesterol levels in children; however, in all likelihood, fiber is equally beneficial at every age. (See p. 167.)

There's a lot of diabetes in my wife's family. Does this mean our children will get diabetes?

Family history plays a role in the development of diabetes, but being overweight is probably the strongest risk factor of all. Reduce your children's risk of Type II diabetes by helping them maintain a healthy weight with a well-balanced diet and regular exercise. Healthy habits you instill in childhood can help keep risk low in the adult years. (See p. 168.)

CHAPTER 13

Food Safety and Additives

Recent serious outbreaks of food poisoning linked to unusual organisms or treatment-resistant strains of common bacteria are warnings we cannot afford to ignore. *Escherichia coli (E. coli)* O157:H7, which has been found in undercooked beef, unpasteurized cider and fruit juices, and contaminated salad greens, among other foods, can lead to hemolytic uremic syndrome (HUS) with kidney failure and death. Infection with campylobacter species, found in undercooked poultry and eggs, can result in painful and bloody diarrhea, as well as Guillain-Barré syndrome, a disease that can cause sudden paralysis in both children and adults. Salmonella, cryptosporidium, and a variety of other bacteria, viruses, and parasites can infiltrate any stage in the food chain and lead to serious illness.

According to government estimates, as many as 80 million Americans may suffer at least one bout of food poisoning, or gastroenteritis, every year. Fortunately, most of us, including healthy older children, can shrug off the uncomfortable symptoms of diarrhea, cramps, and perhaps vomiting in a day or two. However, the very young, the old, and those with chronic diseases may develop complications unless they receive prompt treatment.

Food safety practices on farms, in factories, at packing plants, and during transportation are beyond the control of consumers. In any case, these are relatively minor sources of contamination. The vast majority of cases of food poisoning reported to the Centers for Disease Control and Prevention (CDC) are traced to the way food is handled in homes and food service operations such as cafeterias and caterers. Most episodes could be prevented with simple precautions in the choice, storage, and preparation of food (also see p. 116).

Preventing Foodborne Illness

Those caring for children need to know how to guard against foodborne illnesses. It's never too early to be a good example for children, with proper hand-washing, cleanliness, and careful preparation and storage of food. There are three basic facts to keep in mind when preparing food:

1. **Bacteria rapidly multiply in foods that are lukewarm or kept at room temperature.** Therefore, keep hot foods hot and cold foods cold.

2. **Bacteria are often present in raw foods.** Thoroughly cook foods of animal origin, and thoroughly wash vegetables and fruits that are eaten raw.

3. **Bacteria and viruses are easily transferred from our bodies to food, and from one food to another.** Wash hands frequently and encourage your children to do the same. Never put a spoon used to taste food back into food without washing it. Keep raw foods and cooked foods separate. Wash knives, cutting boards, and other utensils used for preparing one food before reusing for another.

You can reduce your family's risk of foodborne illness by choosing foods in good condition and following a few simple rules for handling, storage, and preparation.

The most common symptoms of food poisoning are:

- Stomach cramps
- Nausea/vomiting
- Diarrhea
- Fever

While similar symptoms may occur in several conditions, food poisoning is the likely cause if two or more members of the household become ill after eating the same dishes. The problem usually clears up if the child avoids eating for a few hours, and takes sips of fluid to replace lost fluid as soon as the vomiting stops. If symptoms are still present after 3 to 4 hours for an infant under 1 year, or 6 to 8 hours for an older child—or if the child appears ill or drowsy, or has bloody or unusually severe diarrhea—call your pediatrician immediately for advice.

Buying Foods

- If you notice unsatisfactory food handling at markets or restaurants, bring it to the manager's attention.
- Check "sell by" and "best before" dates to avoid buying outdated items.
- Don't buy damaged cans or packages.
- Make sure frozen foods are frozen solid, with no ice or water marks indicating the product has been thawed and refrozen.
- Check that foods from the refrigerator case are cold when purchased.
- Inspect eggs and reject any that are dirty, cracked, or unrefrigerated; check freshness dates on the carton.
- Bag meats separately from fresh produce.
- Avoid unpasteurized or "raw" juices and milk, as well as cheese made from unpasteurized or raw milk.

Storing Foods

- Store foods at the correct temperatures; storage at improper temperatures is the most common cause of outbreaks of foodborne illness. Refrigerate or freeze foods as soon as you unpack them. Wrap raw meat, poultry, and fish so they don't come into contact with other foods, especially foods that are eaten raw.
- Keep refrigerated produce in the crisper. Keep other fruits and vegetables at cool room temperature. Protect potatoes from light (a paper shopping bag works well) to guard against the formation of toxic solanine compounds, which are indicated by a green color. Discard potatoes that have turned green and sprouted.
- Store and use cans and packages in date order.
- Store grains and cereals in cupboards or in opaque containers; their vitamin content deteriorates on exposure to light. Similarly, store oils away from light to prevent them from turning rancid.

Preparing Food

- Wash hands for at least 10 to 20 seconds with soap and warm water before preparing foods, and wash again periodically as necessary. If children are helping, tell them to wash long enough to sing their "A, B, Cs" slowly. If you wear rubber gloves, wash your hands with the gloves on.

- Follow the safe-handling labels on prepackaged raw meat and poultry.
- Defrost frozen foods in the refrigerator or under running cold water, not on the countertop or in a bowl of water at room temperature.
- Use separate cutting boards for preparing raw meats and raw produce.
- After using a cutting board or a knife for raw meat, fish, or poultry, wash it with soap and hot water. Rinse the cutting board with a mild bleach solution (1/4 cup of bleach to a gallon of water) before reusing it for any food. Wash plastic cutting boards in the dishwasher, if you have one.
- Cook meat to the recommended temperature and use a meat thermometer if you have difficulty judging when meat is done. Beef and lamb can be eaten rare to medium, provided the internal temperature has reached 140°F, which will kill most bacteria.
- Don't serve hamburgers rare. Unlike germs on the surface of meat, bacteria transferred into ground meat during processing may escape sterilization by the heat of cooking. Cook hamburgers until brown in the center or until the meat thermometer registers 160°F. Reheat ground beef leftovers to 165°F.
- Cook poultry until the thigh joints move easily and the juices run clear; cook poultry pieces such as breasts until the flesh springs back to the touch and no pink color remains.

▷ **MAKING IMPORTED FOODS SAFER**

Despite the vast acreages devoted to food crops in the United States, approximately 38 percent of the fruits and 12 percent of the vegetables Americans eat are grown in other countries. Concern about the rising incidence of germs traceable to imported produce (cyclospora on raspberries from Guatemala, hepatitis A on strawberries from Mexico, cholera in coconut milk from Thailand) led government food authorities to devise a new method of inspecting production sites abroad just as thoroughly as suppliers are monitored in the United States.

According to the new procedures, produce will be banned if farms and processors in the country of origin fail to meet our safety standards. Under the old way of doing things, suspect foods were seized only after they reached the United States port of entry. The far-reaching approach gives the Food and Drug Administration (FDA) the authority to oversee the growing, processing, shipping, and selling of all foods intended for the American market. It covers all agricultural practices, including the use of pesticides, manures and fertilizers, and water for irrigation.

The World Health Organization estimates that for every reported case of foodborne illness worldwide, as many as 350 go unreported. By improving food growing and handling abroad, the new system may reduce the incidence of foodborne illness not only in the United States but also in other countries.

- If you stuff poultry, cook it immediately or, better yet, bake the stuffing in a separate dish.
- Cook pork until no pink color remains, to prevent the spread of trichinosis parasites.
- Rinse salad greens—including prepackaged, prewashed salads—in at least two changes of water.
- Refrigerate leftovers as soon as possible, no longer than 2 hours after serving, to cut down on the time during which bacteria can multiply.

Getting Rid of Pesticides

Regular monitoring of commercial food sources by the Food and Drug Administration (FDA) shows that pesticides are almost always well below the highest levels legally allowed. However, it's a good idea to wash fruits and vegetables to get rid of any residues.

- Wash food in a large amount of cold or tepid tap water.
- Scrub with a brush if necessary, preferably under running water.
- Discard the outer leaves of leafy vegetables, such as lettuce and cabbage.
- When present in foods of animal origin, pesticides tend to be concentrated in the fatty tissues; therefore, trim all visible fat from meat and trim fat and skin from poultry.

Measures to Improve City Water Supplies

Prompted by a major outbreak of illness caused by the parasite cryptosporidium in Milwaukee tap water in 1993, the Environmental Protection Agency revised the requirements for monitoring filtration plants and tightened the standards for turbidity, or cloudiness, in public water systems. For example, the maximum allowable level was reduced by 80 percent between November 1997 and November 1998, and measures to reduce it even further are in progress. In addition, studies are being conducted to determine how often waterborne illness occurs.

Water supplies in the United States are not routinely tested for individual parasites, bacteria, or viruses. Instead, water authorities operate on the assumption that routine filtration and chlorination will reduce microorganisms to a safe level. However, chlorination does not kill cryptosporidium, and the parasite can pass through filtration systems that are not functioning properly. This seems to be what happened in Milwaukee.

If you are concerned about the quality of your local supply, you may prefer to boil drinking water for 5 minutes or buy bottled water until you are assured that the tap water is safe.

> ▶ **RECYCLE SENSIBLY**
>
> Recycling is praiseworthy but should not be carried to extremes. It's not a good idea, for instance, to turn plastic bread bags or other branded plastic bags inside out and use them to store food or pack lunches. The inks used to print the bags can contain lead, which may leach into food. When bags are used as intended, with the printing on the outside, there is no risk to health.

Mercury and Fish

Mercury is released in the form of gas from the earth's crust and oceans or as an industrial by-product. It dissolves in water, where it is transformed by bacterial action into methyl mercury, a more toxic form. When fish absorb methyl

Any animal protein eaten raw or only partly cooked is more likely to cause illness than thoroughly cooked food. When it comes to fish and seafood, the main sources of such illness are bacteria and viruses in water polluted by human waste. There are also harmful marine bacteria that are unrelated to human pollution. They are commonly found in fish and shellfish taken from estuaries, where seas and rivers mingle. In addition, both freshwater and saltwater fish may be colonized by parasites that can transfer to human hosts unless destroyed by freezing or thorough cooking. In susceptible people—especially children, the elderly, and those with chronic illnesses or immune disorders—disease-causing organisms from raw or undercooked fish can cause serious illness. Children should not eat raw fish and shellfish, including dishes prepared like ceviche, which uses soaking in an acidic citrus marinade to "cold cook" the protein.

mercury from the water and from feeding on smaller life-forms, the metal builds up in their tissues. The larger the fish, the greater the intake and buildup. In humans, mercury poisoning can damage the brain and nervous system.

Although contamination is widespread, methyl mercury levels don't reach the FDA limit for human consumption of one part per million (ppm) except in a very few species, such as shark, swordfish, and the large tuna sold as steaks and sushi. The smaller tuna used for canning have much lower levels. Freshwater fish may have high mercury levels, especially in areas where environmental levels are high. The FDA recommends that sport fishers check with state or local government offices for up-to-date information about mercury and other contaminants in local waters and fish. Cooking does not reduce mercury content. Women who are pregnant or planning pregnancy shouldn't eat swordfish or tuna steaks more than once a month, because it's not known what effect low levels of mercury may have on a developing fetus. Those who are nursing may eat a 7-

ounce serving of swordfish, tuna, or other large fish species at the head of the food chain twice a week without exposing their babies to risk. There's no risk of methyl mercury poisoning from eating the top-selling species, which include canned

▷ ADDITIVES THAT ENRICH AND FORTIFY

Additives used for enriching and fortifying foods are particularly beneficial. Enrichment restores essential nutrients that are lost during the processing of raw materials. For example, white flour and rice are enriched with B vitamins that are removed when the grains are milled. As a public health measure, certain foods are fortified with important nutrients to make sure people consume enough to stay healthy. Vitamin D, for example, is added to milk, vitamin A to margarine, and iron and folic acid to flours and cereals.

tuna, shrimp, pollock, salmon, cod, catfish, clams, crabs, and scallops. If you have questions about methyl mercury or other fishy issues, call the 24-hour FDA seafood hotline: 800-FDA-4010.

Additives

Food additives, properly used, allow us to enjoy a variety of wholesome foods in every season. Many people, wary of additives, believe that they are toxic chemicals brewed up in laboratories. Such fears are groundless. The great majority of the 3,000 or so additives allowed by the FDA are foods or normal ingredients of foods. Additives help keep our food healthful in at least five important ways:

- They retard spoilage.
- They improve or maintain nutritional value.
- They make breads and baked goods rise.
- They enhance flavor, color, and appearance.
- They keep flavors and textures consistent.

Additives listed on food labels under their chemical names seem less intimidating when you know their everyday equivalents. For example, salt is sodium chloride, vitamin C is ascorbic acid, and vitamin E is alpha-tocopherol. Not every additive has a familiar name, but it's reassuring to remember that all food is made up of chemicals, just as our bodies are. Regulations known as Good Manufacturing Practices (GMP) limit the amounts of additives that may be used in foods. Manufacturers use only as much of an additive as is needed to achieve the desired result.

The additives most widely used are salt, sugar and corn syrup, vitamin C, vitamin E, and butylated hydroxyanisole (BHA) and butylated hydroxytoluene (BHT). These substances prolong

▷ **ADDITIVES DON'T APPEAR TO INFLUENCE HYPERACTIVITY**

Several years ago, Dr. Benjamin Feingold, a pediatric allergist, claimed that the behavior of hyperactive children improved dramatically when they followed a diet that eliminated additives, including artificial colors and flavors, as well as naturally occurring salicylates in fruits and vegetables. When tested scientifically, the Feingold diet had no favorable effect. Some children, however, appeared to benefit from the extra parental attention. In other cases, belief in the diet's efficacy seemed to bring about an improvement similar to the placebo effect sometimes seen with medical treatments. In one study, the behavior of a small group of children with more severe hyperactivity changed for the worse when they were given food spiked with huge doses of artificial colors. However, the doses were many times greater than children would normally consume, and the findings, therefore, do not apply to usual situations.

Nevertheless, it is possible that a child may be unusually sensitive to a particular ingredient or food. If you are convinced there's a connection between your child's behavior and his diet, talk to your pediatrician, who may perform sensitivity testing or recommend cutting out an offending food and finding alternative sources if essential nutrients are involved (also see Chapters 14 and 15).

According to FDA estimates, about 1 person out of every 100 has allergic symptoms after exposure to sulfites, chemical additives widely used in the food industry. Asthma adds to the risk; sulfites cause serious symptoms in about 5 percent of people with asthma.

Sulfites are added to prolong the shelf life of many fruits, vegetables, and shellfish; to halt the growth of bacteria in wines; and to whiten food starches and condition dough. They are also used as preservatives in some medications. Although once freely allowed under the FDA category of "generally regarded as safe," sulfite use has been more closely regulated in the past dozen years after being linked to numerous health problems, including allergic symptoms ranging in severity from hives and difficulty breathing to fatal anaphylactic shock. While sulfites are indeed harmless to the great majority, they can cause potentially life-threatening reactions in people with asthma and others who are sensitive to the compounds. Scientists haven't yet determined the smallest amount needed to trigger a reaction. Current methods cannot detect sulfite concentrations below 10 parts per million (ppm) in food, although many experts believe that a sulfite-sensitive person may experience symptoms at even lower concentrations. To reduce the risk, the FDA has imposed the following restrictions:

- Sulfites may not be used on fruits and vegetables intended to be eaten raw, such as in supermarket produce departments or restaurant salad bars.
- Product labels must list sulfites that are present in concentrations of 10 ppm or higher, or any sulfites that have been used in processing, regardless of the concentration. In addition, the labels must specify the purpose for which sulfites were used.

If you suspect that exposure to sulfites has triggered hives, chest tightness, difficulty breathing, or other symptoms in your child, call your pediatrician to determine whether a sensitivity is present (also see Chapter 15).

shelf life, stop fats and oils from turning rancid, and prevent discoloration and changes in texture. Additives are also used in packing materials and must be approved for this purpose.

Nitrites and Nitrosamines

Nitrites are chemicals used to cure meats such as bacon and ham and prevent the growth of *Clostridium botulinum,* the bacterium that causes botulism. Nitrites are nothing new; they've been used in one form or another for at least a couple of thousand years. After they reach the digestive tract, some of these chemicals are transformed into nitrosamines, which are potentially carcinogenic, or cancer causing. To keep the risk as low as possible, meat processors are allowed to use only the lowest amount of nitrites needed to stop *C. botulinum.* In addition, cured meats, by law, must contain vitamin C, an antioxidant that blocks the formation of nitrosamines.

Vaccines are made with additives that may be suspending fluids, stabilizers, and preservatives, or adjuvant chemicals that enhance the vaccines' efficacy. Antibiotics are added to prevent the growth of bacteria in cultures, the broths from which vaccines are made. Penicillin is no longer used for this purpose because some people are sensitive to it. Sulfites sometimes are used as preservatives in vaccines; your pediatrician will use an alternative product when immunizing a child who is asthmatic or known to be sensitive to sulfites. A few vaccines are stabilized with monosodium glutamate (MSG), the same MSG used as a flavor enhancer in Asian foods and many commercial food products. In unusually sensitive people, MSG may induce the symptoms of so-called "Chinese restaurant syndrome." These include severe headache, facial flushing, pain, and a feeling of pressure in the chest. If your child has these symptoms, consult your pediatrician to find out whether they are linked to MSG consumption. The amounts of chemical additives in vaccines are so small that they are unlikely to provoke a serious allergic reaction. Still, if you have any concerns about your child's immunizations, or if the child has ever had a reaction following a shot, bring the issue to your pediatrician's attention. Traces of egg protein may be found in vaccines made with chicken eggs. Children who are allergic to eggs should be immunized with vaccines made by other techniques (also see p. 199).

Nutritionists recommend that cured meats be consumed only in moderation, to limit the amount of saturated fats in the diet and to limit exposure to nitrosamines. In addition, a dose of vitamin C in the form of a glass of citrus juice at the same meal may inhibit nitrosamine formation.

Facts About Trans Fats

Nutrition experts have long encouraged consumers to replace saturated fats—animal fats and others that stay firm at room temperature—with unsaturated vegetable oils. To create an acceptable substitute for butter, which is a saturated fat, unsaturated liquid fats are hydrogenated so they will stay firm and resist spoilage through oxidation. Once hydrogenated, these fats are called trans fats and appear to take on not only the

firmness but perhaps other, less desirable properties of butter as well. Mounting evidence suggests that trans fats adversely affect blood cholesterol levels, as butter does, and may contribute to coronary heart disease and, in women, breast cancer.

Experts caution, however, that we should not leap to the conclusion that butter is better. A substantial decrease in coronary heart disease over the past 30 years is partly due to the substitution of unsaturated vegetable fats—including trans fats—for saturated fats. Switching from trans fats back to saturated fats such as butter, lard, and tallow, they warn, would be jumping from the frying pan into the deep-fat fryer. The experts emphasize that new findings offer opportunities to reduce the risk of disease even further. Keep reducing your intake of saturated fats, they say, and at the same time, cut

One of the goals of scientists involved in biotechnology is the production of plants with improved resistance to diseases and pests, enabling farmers to harvest crops with much lower residues of herbicides and pesticides. These plants will satisfy consumers' demands for both high-quality produce and lower levels of synthetic chemicals.

down on your trans fat intake by using liquid oils and soft tub margarines.

There is a strong consumer push for food labels that indicate what proportion of fat content is trans fats. Some manufacturers, recognizing the importance of this information, are voluntarily including it in their advertising. With this information, consumers can note their intake of trans fats correctly in the "saturated" column of their lipid ledger, instead of among the unsaturated oils.

Fat Substitutes

To guard against the health risks linked to long-term consumption of a high-fat diet, all Americans older than 2 are urged to limit their fat intake to 30 percent or less of daily calories, and to keep saturated fat to no more than one third of total fat, or 10 percent of calories. The period between ages 2 and 5 years is one of gradual transition to a low-fat diet. Food producers have responded to the fat reduction trend by developing reduced-fat and nonfat products that often contain fat substitutes.

The FDA allows egg-white- and dairy-pro-tein-based fat substitutes as generally regarded as safe, or GRAS, meaning that they can be used without restriction in food manufacturing. The agency permits more limited use of a newer, sucrose polyester fat substitute. Unlike the earlier products, this one provides no calories at all. It is undigestible; it passes through the digestive tract but cannot be absorbed. In a few people, it can cause a stool-softening effect. Since frequent consumption could deplete the body of fat-soluble vitamins, vitamins A, D, E, and K are added to the product.

Bioengineered Foods

Bioengineering has pushed farmers beyond the age-old practice of selective breeding, whereby one animal or plant strain was crossed with a related one to bring out desirable characteristics and suppress less useful ones. Now, scientists can manipulate genes and create new strains out of unrelated species. Foods, ingredients, and additives produced by bioengineering must meet the

ORGANIC: MEAN WHAT YOU SAY

At the end of 1997 the Department of Agriculture proposed relaxed standards for organic food production, allowing the use of up to 20 percent nonorganic livestock feeds, inclusion of genetically engineered and irradiated foods, and composting with possibly contaminated municipal sludge. After objections by consumers and growers alike, the government withdrew the proposals for revision in keeping with traditional views on what constitutes an organic product.

same FDA safety standards as traditional products. The total acreage of bioengineered crops is still small, but it represents a growing practice.

Food producers are responsible for ensuring that the foods they sell are safe, and the FDA has the authority to remove a food from the market if it poses a risk to public health.

One area of concern related to the transfer of genetic material is the possibility that proteins introduced from one food into another could cause allergic reactions in people sensitive to the first food. For example, a tomato bred to produce a protein normally found in peanuts could cause potentially life-threatening symptoms when eaten by someone allergic to peanuts. For this reason, the FDA requires clear scientific proof of safety from developers working with foods to which people are commonly allergic, such as milk, eggs, wheat, fish, tree nuts (e.g., walnuts, pecans), and legumes (beans, peanuts). It's impossible to predict allergic reactions to proteins derived from plants or other sources if they are not recognized causes of allergy. Nevertheless, scientists can test a bioengineered protein to see whether its structure resembles that of a known allergen. If it does, further tests show whether an allergic cross-reaction is likely.

Organic Foods

Many people prefer to buy organic produce and meat out of concerns for their health and the environment (also see Chapter 14). Purchasers generally assume that foods marketed as "organic" have been grown without synthetic fertilizers and pesticides, and have not been treated with antibiotics, hormones, or synthetic additives such as dyes and preservatives. Even foods raised organically, however, may contain pesticides and other contaminants carried by wind, water, or soil residues. In addition, while free of certain contaminants, organic products are not necessarily more nutritious or more flavorful than other foods. Retailers generally demand higher prices for organic foods, but such produce may spoil faster because it is not treated against insects and bacteria.

Irradiation

Irradiated food is exposed to low levels of X-rays and other forms of ionizing radiation. The process does not make food radioactive, but it kills molds, bacteria, and insects that cause spoilage. It can delay the ripening of fruits, thus extending their shelf life, and it inhibits sprouting of potatoes, onions, garlic and other foods, so they stay fresh longer.

Though consumers have been slow to accept irradiation of food, experts believe it may be a safer means of preservation than many additives. Resistance to irradiated foods seems to be based on persistent but groundless fears of nuclear fallout and radiation sickness. The FDA, which classes irradiation as an additive, allows its use in wheat, flour, potatoes, spices, and many fresh foods. Products that have been irradiated must be labeled and must bear an international symbol.

Avoiding Food Hazards

For children and adults alike, it's good to eat a wide variety of foods. Not only does variety promote a healthful intake of nutrients, but it also lowers the risk of exposure to potentially harmful substances that may be concentrated in one or two foods.

It's not unusual for one or another of my children to have a bout of vomiting and diarrhea after eating something. How can I tell when it's more serious than a touch of food poisoning?

If symptoms are still present after 3 to 4 hours for an infant under 1 year, or 6 to 8 hours for an older child—or if the child appears ill or drowsy, or has bloody or unusually severe diarrhea—call your pediatrician immediately for advice. (See p. 174.)

I'm not sure how long I need to wash my hands to get them really clean for food preparation.

Wash your hands for at least 10 to 20 seconds with soap and warm water before preparing foods, and wash again periodically as necessary. (See p. 173.)

What's the difference between an enriched food and a fortified one?

Enrichment puts back essential nutrients that are lost during the processing of raw materials. White flour and rice are enriched with B vitamins that are lost when the grains are milled. As a public health measure, certain foods are fortified with important nutrients to make sure people consume enough to stay healthy. These nutrients, such as vitamin D in milk and iron in flours and cereals, are not usually present In the food to begin with. (See p. 177.)

With all the new bioengineered foods coming onto the market, who is overseeing safety, especially for people who are allergic to certain foods?

One concern related to bioengineering is the possibility that proteins introduced from one food into another could cause allergic reactions in people sensitive to the first food. For this reason, the FDA requires proof of safety from developers working with foods to which people are commonly allergic. It's impossible to predict allergic reactions to proteins if the sources are not recognized causes of allergy. Still, scientists can test a bioengineered protein to see if it resembles a known allergen. If it does, further tests can show whether a cross-reaction is likely. (See p. 181.)

Does irradiating food make it radioactive?

Experts believe irradiation may be a safer means of preserving food than many additives. The process does not make food radioactive or change it in any way. However, consumers have been slow to accept irradiated foods on the basis of groundless fears of nuclear fallout and radiation sickness. (See p. 182.)

CHAPTER 14

Alternative Diets and Supplements

Maria Baretta took great pride in serving her family the tasty Italian dishes she had learned from her mother and grandmothers. She looked forward to continuing the tradition by teaching her 12-year-old daughter, Anita, the fine art of Italian cooking. Those plans came to a screeching halt when Anita announced that she was becoming a vegetarian, largely because of her concern for animals, plus the fact that her best friend had also decided to become a vegetarian.

"At first, I refused to take her seriously," Maria recalls. "I continued to make my favorite meat dishes, but no amount of pleading or threatening could make Anita eat them."

Finally, Maria consulted her pediatrician. She had expected the doctor to agree that Anita's refusal to eat meat was unhealthy. Instead, the pediatrician assured Maria that a vegetarian diet—especially one like Anita's, which included dairy products and eggs—was just as healthful as one centered around meat dishes. The doctor suggested a couple of books on healthy vegetarian diets, and Maria also bought an Italian vegetarian cookbook. Although many of the Barettas' meals still include a meat dish, Maria also now serves vegetarian alternatives. And instead of hurt feelings or angry dinner-time outbursts over Anita's refusal to eat meat, mealtimes in the Baretta household are peaceful again.

People adopt alternative diets for many reasons—cultural, religious, health, ethical, and environmental, to mention a few. The diets themselves range from age-old vegetarianism to short-lived fads. While some alternative diets can be just as healthful as more traditional fare, when it comes to feeding children, special care is needed to make sure they are well nourished.

A Growing Movement

Only a few years ago, many Americans looked upon vegetarianism with suspicion, often mixed with disdain. Today, a vegetarian diet is almost mainstream compared with the many other alternative diets that are being adopted by a growing number of Americans. Many of these diets make outlandish claims, promising everything from painless weight loss to increased brain power or sports ability. When the diet fails to deliver the promised magic, the person is likely to revert to former eating habits or to try the next fad. Obviously, such faddish or overly restrictive alternative diets should not be forced on growing children.

Still, alternative diets can be just as healthful as a mainstream diet. For children, this means that the diet must provide all of the vitamins, minerals, and energy needed for proper growth and development. Any alternative diet that falls short of meeting the basic nutritional needs of children should be modified or avoided. Similarly, a conventional diet that provides lots of meat, fatty foods, and sweets while skimping on vegetables, fruits, and grains and other starches can lead to serious nutritional problems. Regardless of the type of diet you select, you won't go wrong if you follow the basic rules of variety, moderation, and balance (see Chapter 6).

Vegetarian Diets

In general, a vegetarian is a person who eats mostly plant foods and excludes meat, poultry, and fish from the diet. However, there are many shades of vegetarianism, ranging from partial vegetarians, who eat dairy products, eggs, and perhaps fish and/or poultry, to vegans, strict vegetarians who shun all animal products, including milk and eggs (see box, p. 188).

Although some people still worry that a vegetarian diet is unhealthful, numerous studies have found just the opposite: In general, vegetarians have a reduced risk of obesity, heart disease, high blood pressure, Type II (noninsulin-dependent or adult-onset) diabetes, certain digestive disorders, and some cancers. It is not clear, however, whether these health benefits are due solely to following a vegetarian diet or to a combination of other factors that often go hand in hand with a vegetarian lifestyle; for example, abstaining from smoking and alcohol and exercising regularly.

In a policy statement published in 1988, the American Dietetic Association (ADA) addressed many of the issues related to vegetarian diets:

Vegetarian diets are healthful and nutritionally adequate when appropriately planned. Both vegetarian and nonvegetarian diets have the potential to be either beneficial or detrimental to health.

They went on to say that careful planning of vegetarian diets may reduce the risks for some diseases and help to control some conditions, but poorly planned or haphazard diets increase the likelihood of nutritional deficiencies or excesses.

Health Benefits

Diets based mostly on plant foods are low in cholesterol and saturated fats and high in fiber. Most also provide fewer calories than diets loaded with meat and high-fat dairy products. These factors may account for the lower rates among vegetarians of obesity, heart disease, diabetes, gall bladder disease, and certain cancers.

Plant foods also are rich in vitamins, minerals, and other compounds that are called antioxidants, substances that protect body cells against the damage that naturally occurs when the body burns oxygen. Antioxidants are believed to help prevent some of the cell changes that lead to premature aging and cancer.

Vegetarians often point to other benefits unrelated to health. For example, vegetarian diets tend to be less costly than diets that include meat. Pound for pound, beans and grains are much cheaper sources of protein than meat.

There are also important environmental benefits. It takes many more acres of farm land or pounds of grain to produce a pound of meat than it does to produce an equivalent amount of human plant food. Grains are by far the world's leading foodstuff, and the United States leads the world in per capita grain use. But unlike people in other grain-consuming nations, Americans actually eat very little of this grain themselves. Instead, it is fed to animals to produce meat, eggs, and dairy products.

Finally, many people—especially children and adolescents—become vegetarians because of their concern for animals.

Possible Problems

Nutritionists caution that the design of a healthful vegetarian diet for children takes more planning and knowledge about nutrition than does a diet featuring meat and other animal products. The task is relatively easy, however, if the diet allows eggs and/or milk and other dairy products.

But a strict vegetarian diet is another story. This was reflected in the uproar that arose when the late Dr. Benjamin Spock proposed a strict vegan diet for children over the age of 2. Nutritionists and other experts immediately took issue with the proposal, which was contained in Dr. Spock's 1998 revised edition of *Baby and Child Care*. Children who are fed the vegan diet suggested by Dr. Spock must have supplements or fortified foods to replace essential nutrients that are missing in a vegan diet. Special problem areas for vegans include:

- **Calories.** A growing child may not be able to eat enough plant foods to get the energy needed for proper growth and normal activities, especially in early childhood.
- **Protein,** which is needed to build muscle and other body tissue, must be obtained by balancing foods, such as grains and legumes, to get the range of amino acids that make up high-quality, or complete, proteins.
- **Vitamin B$_{12}$,** which can be absorbed only from animal products, must be obtained from supplements or fortified foods.
- **Vitamin D,** which is found in egg yolks, fish and fish liver oil, and fortified milk and butter, may be lacking. The body also makes vitamin D when the skin is exposed to sunlight, but

▷ ORGANIC? NATURAL? HEALTH FOODS?

Although these terms are often used interchangeably, they have different meanings:
- Organic foods are grown without artificial pesticides, fertilizers, or herbicides.
- Organic meat, eggs, and dairy products are obtained from animals that are fed natural feed and are not given hormones or antibiotics.
- Natural foods are free of synthetic or artificial ingredients or additives.
- "Health foods" is a general term that may be applied to natural or organic foods, or to regular foods that have undergone less processing than usual, such as stone-ground whole-grain flours.

There is no evidence that organic, natural, or health foods are any more nutritious or taste better than regular foods. However, the nutritional content varies greatly according to when the food was harvested and how it has been stored or processed. Taste is determined by plant genetics, rather than by whether the crop is organically or conventionally grown. Harvesting and handling also affect taste. A peach or tomato that is picked when it is too green will never develop the full taste of fruit that is allowed to ripen on the tree or the vine.

Although the type of fertilizer may not affect taste or nutrition, it does have an impact on the environment. Many people prefer to pay premium prices for organic foods because their production does not cause environmental damage from pesticides and herbicides, and composted fertilizers help restore soil and are not as damaging to the environment as artificial fertilizers.

children in northern climates may have difficulty getting enough sun.

- **Calcium,** whose best sources are milk and milk products, must be obtained from plant sources or supplements.
- **Zinc,** whose best sources are beef, liver, and yogurt, may be lacking.

Social Issues

Vegetarianism and other alternative diets can be a major source of conflict unless they are a family affair. Even if parents are strict vegetarians, they should allow their child to eat the foods his friends enjoy, such as an occasional hamburger or roast chicken. However, if the entire family follows a vegetarian diet, the child will grow up accepting it as normal and will also be less likely to feel set apart when he eats foods that are different from what his friends enjoy at school or social gatherings.

The example of the Baretta family at the beginning of this chapter is very typical of what happens when a somewhat older child insists on becoming a vegetarian in a meat-eating family. The switch often occurs during adolescence, a time when many families are strained by a teenager's growing independence. Still, children as young as 6 may become lifelong vegetarians when they become sensitive to the relationship between humans and animals.

A 6-year-old patient of Dr. Stern's asked what he was eating. His mother said, "Fish sticks." He had a pet goldfish. "Fish? Like my fish?" he asked.

When his mother said "Yes," he replied: "That's *disgusting*!" He has not eaten fish (or meat) since, and it has been many years since the incident. A child's continued refusal to eat what parents perceive as foods essential for health sets the stage for mealtime conflicts. Very often, the vegetarian child adopts an irritating moral stance: "You may not care about animals [or the environment], but I do!"

Although adolescents of both sexes become vegetarians, the switch is more common among girls, and concern for animals is by far the most common reason that young people shun meat. In contrast, adults are more likely to cite health reasons for adopting vegetarianism or another alternative diet.

▷ **VARIATIONS ON THE VEGETARIAN THEME**

All vegetarian diets allow grains, vegetables, and fruits, but they vary considerably when it comes to animal products.

Partial vegetarian	Diet allows dairy products, eggs, seafood, and perhaps poultry, but not meat and sometimes not poultry.
Lacto-ovo-vegetarian	Diet allows dairy products and eggs, but not meat, seafood, or poultry.
Lacto-vegetarian	Diet allows milk and milk products, but not eggs, meat, seafood, and poultry.
Ovo-vegetarian	Diet allows eggs, but not meat, seafood, poultry, or milk and other dairy products.
Vegan	No animal products: no dairy products, eggs, meat, seafood, or poultry.

Other Alternative Diets

There are dozens of different alternative diets, but they have certain common themes. Most are built upon philosophical, religious, or other personal convictions. Many promise unlikely benefits, such as rapid and painless weight loss or increased brain power. Some are promoted as treatments (usually unproved) for diseases ranging from childhood hyperactivity to cancer.

Because many of these diets eliminate entire groups of foods, they carry a risk of nutritional deficiencies, especially for children. Some of the most popular alternative diets are summarized in the table on page 192, and described in more detail below.

Whole-Foods Diet

This diet is based on the belief that foods should be eaten in their entirety and in as natural a state as possible. The premise is that whole foods provide a balance of nutrients and energy that is lacking in fragmented or processed foods. Thus, eating a whole baked potato with its skin would be preferable to potatoes that are peeled and cut. In addition to fresh fruits and vegetables, other examples of whole foods include unrefined grains, beans and other legumes, seeds, sea vegetables, and eggs. Fragmented foods, such as sugar, flour, polished rice, and peeled vegetables, are avoided as much as possible. When fragmented foods are eaten, they are balanced with complementary fragments to form a whole. Thus, flour might be balanced with wheat germ and bran to mimic what is found in the whole grain.

Although many people who follow a whole-foods diet are vegetarians, some are not. And some animal products, such as fertilized eggs, are whole foods. A soft-shell crab is also considered a whole food because the entire crab—shell and all—is eaten.

Living Foods Diet

This diet is based on the notion that raw foods are more healthful than cooked ones because they contain enzymes that aid in digestion and, more important, contain the "life force" or natural energy of the plant. Proponents of a living foods diet believe that heating foods destroys these enzymes and also changes the molecular structure of food to make it toxic—an assertion that simply is not true. Cooking certainly does not make foods "toxic." And even if foods are eaten raw, the enzymes will be broken down during digestion.

The diet allows all organically grown fruits, vegetables, sprouts, nuts, seeds, grains, and sea vegetables. Grains and seeds may be soaked so that they are soft enough to eat, but they are not cooked. Beverages include fresh juices and coconut milk. This diet is not recommended for children or adolescents, and adults who follow it are likely to need supplements of vitamin B_{12}, iron, calcium, and zinc. Followers also have an increased risk of foodborne illnesses from eating possibly contaminated uncooked foods.

Variations of the living foods diet include sproutarian, a diet based mostly on sprouted seeds and grains, and juicearian, in which the living foods are put through a juicer. These variations have the same shortcomings as the basic living foods diet.

Fruitarian Diet

This is another extreme variation of a living foods diet that is limited to organically grown fruit, seeds, nuts, and grains. The idea is to avoid killing a plant for food. Thus, carrots and other vegetables are excluded because eating the edible part kills the plant. In contrast, picking an apple or peach does not kill the tree. This diet is potentially dangerous for both children and adults; it

The following menus follow the dictates of the various diets, with suggestions for supplements or fortified foods to fill nutritional gaps.

PARTIAL VEGETARIAN

Breakfast
Whole-grain cereal with low-fat or skim milk
Sliced banana
English muffin
Beverage

Lunch
Tomato and mozzarella salad
Vegetarian bean soup
Whole-grain crackers
Fresh fruit
Low-fat milk

Dinner
Mixed green salad
Baked potato with grated Parmesan cheese
Green beans
Poached fish fillet
Frozen yogurt with oatmeal cookie

Snacks
Low-fat milk or yogurt
Air-popped popcorn
Hummus with pita bread
Choice of fresh fruit or raw vegetables

Supplements: None needed; diet provides proper variety and balance of nutrients.

LACTO-OVO-VEGETARIAN

Breakfast
Orange juice or sliced orange
Scrambled egg
Whole-wheat toast
Skim or low-fat milk

Lunch
Minestrone soup
Fruit salad and cottage cheese
Date bread
Low-fat fruit yogurt

Dinner
Chopped vegetable salad
Pasta with marinara sauce
Low-fat cheese and poached pear
Skim or low-fat milk

Snacks
1/2 toasted bagel or bran muffin
Choice of fresh fruit or vegetables

Supplements: None needed; diet provides proper variety and balance of nutrients.

LACTO-VEGETARIAN

Breakfast
1/2 grapefruit
Oatmeal with mixed dried fruit
Skim or low-fat milk

Lunch
Green salad
Vegetarian chili and rice
Skim or low-fat milk

Dinner
Leek and potato soup
Vegetable lasagne made with cheese
Rice pudding made with low-fat milk

Snacks
Whole-grain crackers
Low-fat yogurt
Fresh fruits or vegetables

Supplements: None needed; diet provides proper variety and balance of nutrients.

OVO-VEGETARIAN

Breakfast
Fresh orange
Poached egg
Whole-wheat toast
Calcium-fortified soy milk

Lunch
Lentil salad
Peanut butter sandwich
Fresh fruit

Dinner
Pasta and bean soup
Steamed broccoli
Vegetarian garden burgers
Tofu ice cream with fresh berries

Snacks
Trail mix; soy milk and fresh fruit shake

Supplements: None needed; diet provides proper variety and balance of nutrients.

VEGAN

Breakfast
Calcium-fortified orange juice
Iron-fortified cereal with dates and soy milk
Fresh fruit

Lunch
Spinach and tomato salad
Vegetarian barley and vegetable soup
Applesauce
Calcium-fortified soy milk

Dinner
Fruit cup
Steamed Chinese vegetables and bean sprouts
Red beans and rice
Fresh berries and sorbet

Snacks
Trail mix, fresh fruit, or vegetables
Calcium-fortified orange juice or soy milk

Supplements: Multiple vitamin-mineral pill to provide vitamin B_{12}, iron, extra calcium, and zinc. Extra snacks or servings may be needed to provide adequate calories.

Whole-foods	Diet is based on belief that foods should be eaten in their whole, natural state. Followers include both vegetarians and meat eaters.
Living foods	Diet allows only organic plant foods that are not cooked, heated, pasteurized, or processed.
Macrobiotic	Diet, part of an Eastern philosophic approach to life, is based mostly on locally grown organic grains, vegetables, legumes, sea vegetables, and soups, although seafood and animal products may be eaten occasionally.
Fruitarian	Diet is based mostly on raw and dried fruits, seeds, sprouted seeds and grains, and nuts; excludes processed and cooked foods, vegetables, and all animal products.
Sproutarian	Variation of living foods diet that consists mostly of sprouts.
Juicearian	Variation of living foods diet based mostly on fresh juices.
Feingold	Diet, designed by an allergist to treat hyperactivity, is promoted as a treatment for attention deficit hyperactivity disorder (ADHD).
Crash weight-loss	These are generally restrictive, low-calorie diets designed to produce rapid weight loss, which is usually temporary.

lacks adequate protein, vitamins B_{12} and D, calcium, iron, zinc, and other trace minerals.

Macrobiotic Diets

Closely related to Zen Buddhism, macrobiotic diets are largely vegetarian and rooted in Eastern philosophy. All foods are classified as yin (female) or yang (male), and meals seek to balance these so-called opposing natural forces. Thus, yang foods—meat, seafood, seeds, and grains—are served with yin foods—vegetables, fruits, juices, and dairy foods. An individual diet is tailored to the specific yin or yang needs of the person. If a person falls ill with a yang disease, yin foods in the diet should be increased to try to restore the bal-

ance of yin and yang. In addition, foods should be seasonal, locally grown, and prepared in a specific manner with wooden cooking utensils.

The extreme macrobiotic diets that were popular in the United States during the 1960s created a lot of misunderstanding of macrobiotics and the underlying philosophy. These extreme diets, which are no longer widely practiced, were limited mostly to brown rice and other grains, legumes, and teas. Following such a restrictive diet for very long can cause severe nutritional deficiencies, and some deaths were attributed to these macrobiotic regimens. The traditional macrobiotic diet, however, emphasizes variety and balance, and can be healthful, but it requires time to learn and to prepare.

Folk medicine is filled with dietary remedies to treat various diseases, and research shows that some of these may be helpful. For most medical conditions, however, modern medicines are more effective and easier to control than dietary remedies. Extra caution is needed when using a diet to treat a childhood disorder. Two prominent examples are the ketogenic diet to treat epilepsy and the Feingold diet to treat attention deficit hyperactivity disorder (ADHD).

■ The Ketogenic Diet

This diet is used to treat epileptic seizures that cannot be controlled with medication. It is a low-calorie diet that is made up mostly of high-fat foods—lots of cream, butter, cheese—with a limited amount of protein and vegetables, and no sugar or starch. Studies by Johns Hopkins neurologists show that seizures in 70 percent of children who are put on a ketogenic diet improve, and most can go off the diet in two or three years.

The ketogenic diet is designed to mimic the metabolism that occurs during fasting. Instead of burning mostly glucose for energy, the body is forced to burn mostly fat. Even ancient healers observed that fasting could halt seizures, but fasting is hardly a long-term treatment for epilepsy. Although there are some widely publicized success stories of children whose epilepsy was brought under control by the ketogenic diet, doctors stress that it's not a do-it-yourself solution. The diet must be very carefully structured for the individual child and then followed exactly. It is essential to make sure that the child obtains enough protein. Frequent check-ups are necessary to make sure the child is growing normally and not suffering any adverse effects.

■ The Feingold Diet

This diet, developed by the late Dr. Benjamin Feingold, is designed to treat childhood hyperactivity that may be caused by food allergies. It calls for eliminating all foods that contain artificial colors, flavors, and three common preservatives: BHA, BHT, and TBHQ. Also eliminated are aspirin and foods that contain natural salicylates, compounds found in aspirin. These include apples, apricots, berries, cherries, cucumbers, currants, grapes, green peppers, tomatoes, nectarines, oranges, peaches, plums, prunes, and tangerines, as well as tea and coffee.

If any of these foods contributes to hyperactivity, an improvement should be noted after a few weeks on the diet. To further identify the offending foods, those in the salicylate group can be reintroduced, one at a time, every five or six days. After each food is reintroduced, the child should be watched to see if symptoms recur. If so, the food should be eliminated from the diet. If not, it can be assumed to be safe, and the child can go on to the next food on the list.

Studies have shown that the Feingold diet fails to control hyperactivity. Some parents, however, insist that the diet helps.

Crash Weight-Loss Diets

It seems that every few months, yet another "miracle" weight-loss diet comes along. Although the specifics vary, all promise that you'll quickly and easily shed unwanted pounds. And those who follow these diets for even a few weeks do, indeed, lose weight. But as soon as they stop dieting, the lost weight returns, often with a few extra pounds added. The main reason these diets fail is that they don't address the underlying reason for being overweight: faulty eating habits, lack of exercise, and perhaps hereditary and metabolic factors. So

▷ THE QUESTION OF SUPPLEMENTS

Nutritionists agree that most healthy people—both adults and children—who consume a varied diet based on the Food Guide Pyramid (p. 90) do not need vitamin and mineral supplements. However, millions of Americans persist in taking a daily multiple vitamin pill "to be on the safe side." Although the pill may not be needed, it probably will not do any harm so long as it does not exceed 100 percent of the RDA for any vitamin or mineral.

There are instances, however, in which higher doses of a specific vitamin or mineral may be needed. Children who cannot properly absorb fats in the diet may need supplements of fat-soluble vitamins A, D, E, and K. An adolescent girl with very heavy periods may require extra iron to keep from becoming anemic. Children on a strict vegetarian diet or those with rare metabolic disorders may also need supplements. In such cases, you should rely on your pediatrician to prescribe the nutrient and its dosage.

Serious problems can develop when vitamins or minerals are given in very large amounts, or megadoses. When given in megadoses, vitamins and minerals take on the property of drugs, and like all drugs, they carry a risk of adverse side effects. Unfortunately, many people try to self-treat various conditions—everything from the common cold to childhood mental illnesses—with megadoses of vitamins and minerals. This is referred to as orthomolecular therapy, a term coined by the late Dr. Linus Pauling to describe the treatment or prevention of disease with megadose vitamins.

There have been a number of reports of children with autism, psychoses, hyperactivity, and dyslexia and other learning disorders improving under orthomolecular therapy. Unfortunately, none of these findings have been proved in controlled scientific studies. Indeed, one study of high-dose vitamin therapy to treat hyperactivity found no benefit, but 42 percent of the children were found to have potentially serious nutritional imbalances. So when it comes to giving high doses of any vitamin or mineral, always check with your pediatrician first. Unless your child has a rare nutritional deficiency or a specific disorder, your pediatrician is likely to advise against high-dose vitamins.

when you go off such a diet and return to your normal eating habits, you again gain weight.

There are many types of crash diets; examples include liquid-protein diets, low-carbohydrate diets (e.g., the Atkins, Stillman, and Scarsdale diets), herbal diets, and diets based on one or two foods (e.g., grapefruit or cabbage diets). All of these pose special hazards for children (see Chapter 8), and most doctors do not recommend them for adults, either.

ISSUES PARENTS RAISE ABOUT ALTERNATIVE DIETS

My teenage son has told me he won't eat meat from now on. He's still growing, and I'm concerned that he'll get too little protein if he eats nothing but nuts and berries.
A vegetarian diet can be healthful and nutritionally balanced when based on the Food Guide Pyramid (see p. 90). Your son can get more than enough protein from grains and legumes, especially if his diet includes animal foods such as dairy products and eggs. A vegetarian diet can be economical, too. In fact, pound for pound, grains and beans are much cheaper sources of protein than meat. Regardless of the diet your son adopts, he won't go wrong if he follows the basic rules of variety, moderation, and balance.

Do children on vegetarian diets need supplements to make up for missing nutrients?
Children on properly planned vegetarian diets that include some animal foods—such as eggs, milk and other dairy foods, or fish—are unlikely to need supplements. However, a strict vegan diet that excludes all animal products may be lacking in vitamins B_{12} and D, as well as the minerals calcium and zinc (see p. 187). If your family follows a vegan lifestyle, ask your pediatrician's advice to make sure that your children are getting the full range of nutrients together with the calories they need for growth.

Are organic foods and health foods better for you than regular foods from the market?
There's no evidence that organic, natural, or health foods are more nutritious than regular foods. The nutritional content of food varies according to when it was harvested and how it has been stored or processed. However, many people prefer foods from crops that have been raised without artificial pesticides, fertilizers, and herbicides or—in the case of meat, eggs, and dairy products—from animals raised on natural feed and not given hormones or antibiotics. Many people also prefer to pay more for organic foods because their production causes less damage to the environment. (See p. 187.)

CHAPTER 15

Is My Child Allergic?

Shortly after his fourth birthday, Leshawn's sweet temperament turned sour. He was often irritable and complained of a stomachache. His appetite dropped off and he frequently had loose, watery stools and a lot of gas. Because Leshawn usually developed the symptoms about an hour after meals and didn't have any other problems, such as a fever or headache, his mother wondered if he might have an allergy. However, she couldn't trace the symptoms back to any one food. After listening to her description of the symptoms, Leshawn's pediatrician sent him for a simple breath test that confirmed his suspicions. Leshawn was not allergic. His symptoms were caused by lactose intolerance, an inability to digest the natural sugar in milk and some other dairy products. Symptoms followed meals because he usually drank milk at mealtimes. The pediatrician referred Leshawn and his mother to a registered dietitian, who guided them in the use of lactase enzyme supplements, which break down lactose to an easily digested form. She also suggested the use of lactose-free milks, and other dairy foods with reduced lactose levels. In addition, she suggested non-dairy foods as alternative sources of calcium.

Food allergies are blamed for symptoms and disorders ranging from irritability, hyperactivity, and gastro-intestinal discomfort to asthma and chronic fatigue syndrome. However, true food allergies are quite rare, and affect no more than 2 out of 100 people. Almost half of all children who develop food allergies before age 3 eventually grow out of them.

Allergy Versus Adverse Reactions

Most symptoms caused by foods in young children are not allergic reactions, but are called "adverse reactions to foods." In an allergy, the immune system mistakenly tries to defend the body against certain food proteins as if they were invading germs. By contrast, an adverse reaction can produce symptoms similar to those of allergy, but usually does not involve the immune system.

These reactions most commonly occur in the first year of life and disappear by the time the child is 3 years old. Approximately one third of all children have such reactions. Digestive tract symptoms such as diarrhea, vomiting, spitting up, and colic are the most frequent, followed by skin rashes and itching, runny nose or congestion, and wheezing. In most cases, the immune system is not involved and other mechanisms are responsible. Other adverse reactions can be related to individual responses to additives and ingredients. Typical examples are rashes caused by sensitivity to artificial flavors and colors. Some reactions, such as wheat sensitivity in celiac disease, are lifelong conditions.

Food Allergy

In an allergic person, the immune system reacts to protein in a specific food. On exposure to the food, the body produces an antibody (immuno-globulin) to the protein. Substances that cause allergies are called allergens. The more antibody the body makes, the more severe the symptoms.

Anaphylaxis is a rare, serious allergic reaction. Symptoms of anaphylaxis include:

- Swelling in the mouth and throat.

- Difficulty in breathing.

- Collapse/shock.

Anaphylaxis is a life-threatening emergency and requires immediate medical attention. Call the Emergency Medical Services (911) at once. Food allergy can kill.

It may take weeks, months, or years before antibody builds up, but once it does, a repeat exposure to the food triggers the release of histamine, causing allergic symptoms ranging from runny nose, itchy eyes, diarrhea, and rash to wheezing; swelling of the lips, tongue, or mouth; itching; and tightness in the throat. Symptoms may appear immediately—that is, within a few minutes and up to 2 hours after eating—or after 2 hours but usually in less than 72 hours.

The only way to manage allergies is to strictly avoid the offending food. Although allergies cannot be cured, almost half of children younger than 3 with food allergies outgrow them by about age 7, and 95 percent of those with cow's milk allergy outgrow it by age 3. Allergies to foods such as nuts and shellfish are more likely to persist for life. Children whose symptoms develop after age 3 are less likely to grow out of the problem. Fortunately, a child is rarely allergic to more than one food.

Common Causes of Allergy

Cow's milk is the most common cause of food allergy among young children. Cow's milk allergy affects 2 or 3 out of every 100 young children. Fortunately, most outgrow the allergy and can tolerate milk by age 4. If your breastfed baby develops recurrent diarrhea, spitting up, and gas after you have consumed milk or other dairy foods, eliminating such foods from your diet may relieve the baby's symptoms. Be sure to seek your pediatrician's advice and find alternative sources of calcium as long as you are breastfeeding. If your bot-

▷ **FOODS AND INGREDIENTS TO AVOID IF YOUR CHILD IS ALLERGIC TO MILK**

Buttermilk	Cream	Powdered milk
Calcium caseinate	Evaporated milk	Sherbet (if made with milk)
Casein	Ice cream, ice milk, frozen yogurt	Sodium caseinate
Cheese, cottage cheese	Margarine	Whey
Condensed milk	Milk chocolate	Yogurt
Cow's milk	Milk solids	

tle-fed infant appears to be allergic to cow's milk formula, your pediatrician may recommend another formula such as one made with hydrolyzed protein. Soy formula should not be used because more than half of all children who are allergic to cow's milk protein are also allergic to soy protein. For babies who have difficulty tolerating the usual kinds of formulas, pediatricians generally recommend a formula made with predigested protein that is unlikely to trigger a reaction.

When you introduce solid foods, check labels to make sure that products are free of cow's milk protein, which may appear under various names (see box on previous page). Tell your child's caregivers about the seriousness of the allergy and the importance of avoiding products containing cow's milk protein.

Eggs are another common allergen. Specifically, it's the protein-rich egg white that is allergenic. Egg white should not be given to a child younger than 12 months, to reduce the likelihood of triggering an allergy. However, most infants can eat egg yolks without a problem. When reading labels, avoid foods that contain albumin, globulin, ovomucin, or vitellin, which are all extracted from eggs. Give egg substitutes only if your pediatrician advises it; while such products are cholesterol free, they are not egg free. In very rare cases, egg allergy may cause a reaction to the MMR (measles, mumps, and rubella) and flu vaccines because eggs are used to make them. Such reactions have not been seen in infants younger than one year. If you have a strong family history of allergies, or your child is severely allergic to eggs, check with your pediatrician before your baby receives the MMR immunization.

Wheat allergy (not to be confused with gluten intolerance; see p. 202) is the most common grain allergy. It's best to delay giving wheat until after

▷ **REACTIONS TO DYES AND PRESERVATIVES**

Life-threatening reactions may be triggered in sensitive people by food dyes—such as tartrazine yellow and cochineal (a red coloring extracted from insects)—and preservatives, especially sulfites, which are used to prolong the shelf-life of some fruits and vegetables, shellfish, and certain medications, as well as to whiten food starches and condition dough (see Chapter 13). Foods containing such additives should not be given to children with asthma or to young children with a family history of allergies.

your baby has successfully managed rice and oats. After about 6 to 8 months of age, it's probably safe. But if anyone in your family has an allergy, the chances are increased that your infant will also be allergic. Aside from breads and baked goods, wheat can be found in a wide variety of foods including salad dressings, processed (American) cheese, and breaded fish sticks and chicken nuggets. Wheat is also a hidden ingredient in many commercial food products such as canned soups and stews. Read labels carefully. If you want to offer breads and cereals but avoid wheat, try pure oat or rye breads; corn tortillas; oat, rice, or rye crackers; and cereals made with oats, corn, or rice.

Soy allergies sometimes emerge when an infant is given a soy-based formula. If your child is allergic to soy, read all food labels carefully, because soy products are used in many processed foods. Code words that may indicate the presence of soy include textured vegetable protein, emulsifiers, flavorings, stabilizers, lecithin, shortening, and vegetable oil.

► FOOD ALLERGY SYMPTOMS IN INFANTS

Signs and symptoms of a possible food allergy in infancy include the following:

- Skin rash/eczema.

- Vomiting most or all food after feeding.

- Loose, watery stools eight or more times a day.

- Bloody diarrhea.

Peanuts can provoke such a sensitive allergic reaction in some children that even a kiss from someone who has eaten peanut butter can set it off. Because peanuts can be found in unlikely foods, including chili and chocolate chips, it's essential to read labels. Peanuts are actually legumes from the pea and bean family, not true nuts. Therefore, some children who are allergic to peanuts have no problems with tree nuts such as pecans and walnuts. Similarly, those who are allergic to tree nuts may tolerate peanuts.

Corn allergy, although rare, can show up in infancy if a baby is given a formula that contains corn oil. It's relatively easy to avoid sources such as corn-based cereals. However, corn turns up in many less obvious foods and additives in the form of a dusting of cornmeal on breads, muffins, and pasta; high-fructose corn syrup added to juices and soft drinks; the caramel widely used to color foods; dextrin, dextrose, lactic acid, and maltodextrins; and mannitol and sorbitol, the nonabsorbable sweeteners used in gums and other sugarless foods.

Citrus fruits occasionally cause allergies or adverse reactions. Some pediatricians advise waiting until after age one before introducing citrus juice, to lessen the risk of triggering an allergy. If your pediatrician advises waiting, check all labels carefully; citrus juices are frequently among the ingredients of commercial juice mixtures and punches.

Diagnosing Food Allergies

Diagnosis of food allergies is controversial and can be tricky. Children are most likely to have adverse reactions to food in their first year and less likely to do so after age 3. However, allergies may appear at any age.

If your child has symptoms that occur anywhere from a few minutes to 72 hours after consumption of a particular food, or that cannot be explained, check with your pediatrician.

As you wean your infant to solid foods, play it safe by introducing no more than one food at a time every 2 or 3 days. This makes it easier to trace the cause of any symptoms that may occur.

If symptoms suggesting food allergy appear, the

► COMMON SYMPTOMS OF FOOD ALLERGY

At any age, food allergy may trigger:

- Respiratory tract symptoms such as runny nose, sneezing, wheezing, and coughing.

- Gastrointestinal symptoms such as bloating, stomachache, cramping, nausea, and diarrhea.

- Skin symptoms such as hives, a rash, and itching.

If the symptoms are triggered by allergy, your child will not have a fever.

COMMON ALLERGY TRIGGERS

> Any food has the potential to trigger either an allergy or an intolerance, although certain foods are more likely than others to cause problems. The most common food allergy triggers are cow's milk and other dairy products, egg whites, poultry, seafood, wheat, nuts, soy, and chocolate.

suspect food is eliminated from the diet for 2 weeks, or until symptoms lessen. When symptoms cannot be traced to a particular food, your doctor may prescribe a diet similar to the allergy diet on page 202, which allows only foods that are unlikely to cause reactions. If your child has symptoms that suggest a food allergy but the cause is not clear, your pediatrician will probably provide a referral to a pediatric allergist for skin or blood tests. Even though a child may outgrow allergy symptoms, the response to the skin-prick test usually remains positive. Skin and blood tests indicate the presence of allergy in about half of all cases.

Food Intolerance

A food intolerance is an abnormal, nonallergic response to a food or additive. Two of the most common such responses are lactose intolerance and gluten intolerance. People who are lactose intolerant, like 4-year-old Leshawn, produce insufficient amounts of lactase, the enzyme needed to digest the natural sugar in milk. Most people of Asian, African, and Native American ancestry gradually lose the ability to digest lactose starting at about age 4 or 5. In contrast, those of

Northern European descent can usually digest milk and other dairy foods throughout their lives.

Undigested lactose is broken down by bacteria in the large intestine, producing gas and discomfort. Symptoms such as cramping, bloating, flatulence, and diarrhea occur about 30 minutes to 2 hours after consumption of lactose. The diagnosis can be confirmed by measuring the amount of hydrogen in a person's breath after consumption of a lactose-containing food.

Lactose intolerance is uncomfortable, but—unlike some allergies—it is not life threatening. Lactose-intolerant people vary greatly in their

LACTOSE IN COMMERCIAL FOODS

> Milk is the only natural source of lactose, but the milk sugar is often added to commercial products such as the following:
>
> - Bread and other baked goods
> - Candies and snacks
> - Instant potatoes, soups, and breakfast drinks
> - Margarine
> - Medications (as a filler)
> - Mixes for pancakes, biscuits, and cookies
> - Nondairy creamers
> - Nonkosher lunch meats and hot dogs
> - Processed breakfast cereals
> - Salad dressings

This diet allows only foods that are unlikely to cause reactions.

Foods and Beverages Allowed	Foods to Avoid
Lamb	Milk
Rice	Tea
Rice wafers	Coffee
Rice cereals	Cola
Blueberries	Soft drinks
Loganberries	Chewing gum
Pears	All medications, unless prescribed
Pineapple	by a physician
Artichokes	All foods not listed in first column
Beets	
Celery	
Lettuce	
Parsnips	
Salt	
Spinach	
Sugar (cane or beet)	
Water	
Any vegetable oil, but not margarine	

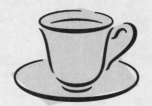

ability to digest lactose. Many can eat at least some yogurt and cheese, because most of the lactose is broken down in processing. Some can drink a little milk as long as it is accompanied by food. If a child cannot drink milk or eat dairy products, it is important to make sure that the diet includes plenty of calcium.

There are plenty of choices for those who are lactose intolerant. Lactose-free milk and dairy products are available; chewable lactase supplements can be taken before lactose-containing foods are eaten to aid lactose digestion; and lactase enzyme drops can be added to regular milk to predigest the lactose.

Nondairy options that are lactose-free include milks made from soy, rice, oats, or almonds, in addition to tofu beverages; however, most have less calcium than real milk. You can also replace dairy cheese with cheese made from rice, tofu, almond, or soy. Bear in mind, however, that while these products are lactose-free, some contain milk proteins, which are off-limits for those who are allergic to milk.

Temporary lactose intolerance may follow a bout of infectious diarrhea in a baby. The symptoms disappear as the condition clears up. Your pediatrician may recommend a lactose-free formula for a week or two.

Gluten enteropathy, also called celiac disease and gluten intolerance, is an inability to tolerate gluten, a protein found in many grains (also see Chapter 7). Exposure to gluten damages the folds of the small intestinal lining, which prevents the absorption of many nutrients, including protein, carbohydrates, fats, and fat-soluble vitamins. The cause of gluten enteropathy is not known, but it is thought to be a hereditary abnormality in part of the immune system involving the intestine. Typical symptoms of irritability, diarrhea and/or constipation, and poor growth and weight gain usually appear after an affected baby is introduced to cereal.

The intestinal damage may lead to lactose intolerance and loss of electrolytes. Poor absorption of vitamins may cause complications such as softening of the bones (osteomalacia), rickets, muscle spasms, night blindness, abnormal blood clotting, and anemia. A person with gluten enteropathy must strictly avoid cereals, breads, pasta, and any other foods made with grains containing gluten. Your pediatrician will provide dietary advice and refer your child to a nutritionist for guidance. After a gluten-free diet is established, the intestinal tract begins to repair itself and symptoms subside. However, the diet must be followed for life. If your child eats gluten, the symptoms will recur.

Can Food Allergies Be Prevented?

If allergies run in your family, the chances are higher that your child will have them. However, it's possible to delay or prevent some allergies by eliminating major food allergens from the diets of infants at high risk for allergy and—if they're being breastfed—from their mothers' diets as well. Breastfeeding itself seems to protect against cow's milk allergy. Young children have a greater risk of an allergic reaction when they switch to solid food to supplement breastmilk or formula. In addition to regular cow's milk, it is best to avoid wheat, seafood, and egg whites until about age one, to reduce the risk.

Rice cereal is most often recommended as the first solid food for infants, because rice is gluten

▷ **HIDDEN GLUTEN**

- Alcohol-based flavorings (such as vanilla extract)
- Brown rice syrup
- Canned broth
- Caramel flavor
- Distilled vinegar (an ingredient in condiments such as ketchup, pickles, mayonnaise, salad dressings, and barbecue sauce)
- Flour and cereal products
- Hydrolyzed vegetable protein
- Imitation seafood
- Malt or malt flavoring
- Maltodextrin
- Modified food starch
- Self-basting poultry
- Vegetable gum
- Vegetable protein

The American Academy of Pediatrics recommends the following to prevent or delay food allergies in infants at high risk (such as those with a family history):

- Do not restrict any potentially allergenic foods during pregnancy (however, your doctor may suggest that you avoid some known trigger foods).

- Breastfeed exclusively for the first 6 months or use a low-allergenic formula (no cow's milk or soy protein), as recommended by your pediatrician.

- Eliminate nuts and peanuts from the mother's diet, and possibly eggs and milk.

- Delay the introduction of solid foods until after 4 to 6 months of age.

- Delay the introduction of cow's milk until age 1, eggs until age 2, and peanuts, nuts, and fish until age 3 (nuts should not be given to children younger than 4 except in the form of smooth nut butter spread thin on bread or crackers).

free and less likely than other grains to cause a reaction. As you add other cereals to your baby's diet, check ingredient labels carefully. Some high-protein and mixed-grain cereals contain wheat.

Give your baby just one new food at 2- to 3-day intervals. If symptoms such as diarrhea, rash, or vomiting appear, stop giving the food in question until you've talked to your pediatrician. Follow the recommendations in Chapter 2 for introducing foods and expanding your baby's diet.

Large amounts of fruit or juice can make a baby's stool acidic and irritating to the skin. The resulting painful red rash is sometimes mistaken for an allergic reaction. Cutting down on fruit, and either diluting juice half and half with water or omitting juice altogether may help get rid of the irritation.

Allergies and Hyperactivity

Parents often blame candies and other high-sugar foods when children get unruly. Some insist that sugar triggers hyperactivity. However, when put to the test, the sugar-behavior link does not hold up. In a carefully controlled study of preschool and school-age children, researchers found no effect on behavior or ability to concentrate when sugar intake was far above normal, even among those whom parents identified as "sugar sensitive." Another study found that sugar had the opposite effect to what was expected: When boys whose parents believed them to be sugar reactive were each given a large dose of sugar, they were actually less active than before. Finally, several studies comparing blood glucose levels have found that children with attention deficit hyperactivity disorder (ADHD) have exactly the same response to sugar consumption as normal children do.

A moderate amount of sugar is acceptable as part of a balanced diet. There is no scientific basis for claims that sugar and other sweeteners influence behavior or cause ADHD, even at levels many times higher than in a normal diet.

Special diets for the treatment of hyperactivity are based on the belief that allergies or reactions to foods cause undesirable behavior. The diets typically target artificial additives, sugar, or the commonly allergenic foods (corn, nuts, chocolate, shellfish, wheat). However, no links have been established between foods and behavior. Therefore, the American Academy of Pediatrics does not recommend special diets for the treatment of hyperactivity. If your child behaves oddly or has unusual symptoms after eating a particular food, it will do no harm to avoid it, provided his or her diet includes other choices from the same food group. (Also see Chapters 13 and 14.)

Asthma and Allergies
A family history of any type of allergy increases the risk that a child may have asthma. Children with asthma and food allergies are at increased risk for anaphylaxis, a severe allergic reaction, even when their asthma is well controlled.

For children with known food allergies, especially those who also have asthma, parents should be thoroughly familiar with food ingredients. They should also carry an emergency dose of epinephrine at all times. Epinephrine, a drug that stops or slows down anaphylaxis, is available in spring-loaded self-injectable syringes. Though not a cure, a dose of epinephrine administered soon after symptoms begin should stall severe symptoms long enough to get the necessary medical attention.

Living with a child who has anaphylactic sensitivity to food can be difficult. Young children cannot fully understand the need for dietary restriction, and their older siblings must be taught how serious food allergy is. The food aller-

 FOOD CHALLENGE FOR ALLERGY

If your child has been diagnosed with a food allergy and you want to test whether he has outgrown it, a food challenge should be performed only in your doctor's office—*never at home*—in case a severe allergic reaction occurs.

gen should be eliminated from the home or, where this is impossible, warning stickers should be placed on foods containing the allergen. It is particularly important to inform your child's teachers, friends, fellow students and neighbors about the dangers. Children should be warned never to test whether claims of allergies are true by hiding the allergen in another child's food.

Sulfites, which are used to stop discoloration, overripening, and spoiling, are known to trigger asthma attacks. These additives are found in processed beverages and foods, including fruit juices, soft drinks, cider vinegar, potato chips, dried fruits and vegetables, maraschino cherries, and wines. Numerous reports of allergic reactions—mostly among people with asthma—and of deaths associated with sulfite ingestion have led the FDA to ban the use of sulfites in fresh fruits and vegetables (also see Chapter 13). Sulfites may be used in certain processed foods, provided they are listed on labels when present in quantities higher than 10 parts per million, or when used at all in manufacturing. Processed potatoes and some canned foods may contain sulfites. If your child has asthma or is sensitive to sulfites, be cautious about any processed or prepared food.

What's the difference between a food allergy and an intolerance, like lactose intolerance?

In an allergic person, the immune system reacts to protein in a certain food. In contrast to allergy, the immune system is not involved in a food intolerance. A person with food intolerance usually does not make enough of a certain enzyme required for the digestion of some part of a food. (Also see p. 197)

My 18-month-old has eczema and when our pediatrician tested him, she found he was sensitive to cow's milk. Does this mean he can't eat dairy foods for the rest of his life?

In many cases, children outgrow sensitivities to cow's milk and other foods, often by age 3 or 4. True, lifelong food allergies are quite rare. Ask your pediatrician for guidance about which foods your child should avoid and for how long. (Also see p. 198).

Lots of members of my husband's family are allergic to different foods. Is there any way to lower my baby's risk of being allergic?

If allergies run in the family, the risk is higher than average that your child will also develop allergies. However, it is possible to delay or even prevent some allergies by eliminating common food allergens from the diets of infants at high risk and—if the babies are being breastfed—from the mothers' diets as well. Breastfeeding itself seems to protect against cow's milk allergy so long as the mother avoids drinking cow's milk. Young children have a greater risk of an allergic reaction when they start eating solid foods to supplement breastmilk or formula. To reduce the risk of developing allergies in all infants, it's best to avoid giving them cow's milk, wheat products, seafood, and egg whites until about age one. (Also see p. 203.)

What Caregivers Need to Know: A Checklist

Parents should provide baby-sitters and caregivers with specific instructions about feeding children: not only about what to serve, but also when, where, and how. Most teenage sitters and those new to the household need more details than extended-family members and the usual sitters do. Parents may need to be tactful with older family members, as the practices they are comfortable with do not necessarily suit a new generation.

If you are leaving a picky eater in the care of a sitter, pass on any necessary information out of the child's hearing and avoid giving overly detailed instructions. Many picky eaters will eat without a fuss when sharing a meal with other children or with caregivers. The less attention paid to their demands, the easier meals can be.

For Babies and Young Children

✔ If a new baby-sitter will be caring for infants and toddlers, arrange a time before the actual baby-sitting date for the sitter to visit your home during a meal, to observe and help feed the children. In this way, the sitter will be familiar with the routine before taking on the job alone, the children will be more comfortable with the sitter, and the parents can be more confident that meal-times will go smoothly.

For Infants

✔ If you are breastfeeding, and if you usually express and refrigerate breastmilk for times when you must be away from your baby, show your sitter how to warm the bottles.

✔ For a bottle-fed infant, mix and refrigerate several bottles of formula before going out.

✔ Show the sitter how to warm a bottle by standing it in a pitcher of warm water, and how to flick a few drops on to the wrist to test that the temperature is no hotter than lukewarm.

✔ Warn the sitter never to heat bottles in the microwave.

For Toddlers and Older Children

✔ If the children's food is already prepared and needs only to be heated, leave written instructions about oven temperatures and timing. Show the sitter how to use the oven, microwave, and other appliances.

✔ When you expect the sitter to prepare the meal, leave all the ingredients and utensils ready, together with clear, written instructions.

✔ Let the sitter know exactly what are appropriate finger foods and be clear about those that your child is still too young to manage (see Unsafe for Toddlers, p. 47).

✔ If you prefer that your child not have cookies, candy, and other sugary foods, make sure the sitter is aware of your concerns and provide other choices for treats.

For Children With Special Needs

✔ If your child has a chronic condition that requires a special diet, such as diabetes, cystic fibrosis, or gluten enteropathy (celiac disease), provide written, step-by-step procedures for all meals and snacks. Also provide clear instructions about how to protect a child with cystic fibrosis against excessive salt loss and dehydration in warm weather.

✔ Be sure to leave a list of permitted treats as

well as a list of foods that the child absolutely cannot eat.

✔ If your child has diabetes, leave written instructions about the importance of regular meals and snacks, and what foods may be eaten. Many people have the mistaken impression that children with diabetes can never eat sweets or candy. This is not so. While foods with added sugar should be consumed sparingly, as recommended in the Food Guide Pyramid (p. 90), they are not forbidden for diabetic children. Sweet foods have a place in a balanced and nutritious diet plan. In your written instructions, include a list of allowable exchanges and emphasize that any sugary food the child consumes must be included in the overall carbohydrate allowance for a given meal or snack

✔ In the case of food allergy or sensitivity, go over the list of foods that must be avoided because they may contain the food or ingredient that causes the allergy but in hidden forms.

✔ To help the caregiver to be ready for problems and to be able to find help when necessary, write out a list of symptoms that may be related to food, such as vomiting, diarrhea, wheezing, rash, hives, swelling, and difficulty breathing.

✔ Leave the list of symptoms next to the numbers to call in case of emergency (pediatrician, Poison Center, 911, close neighbor).

For All Children

✔ Give the sitter a written schedule of doses for any medicine your child must take while you are gone, including the times when the medicine should be taken.

✔ Make sure the caregiver knows how to deal with a choking infant and how to perform the Heimlich maneuver for an older child who is choking (see p. 48).

Food-Medication Interactions

Medical treatments can affect the way children digest and absorb food. By the same token, what youngsters eat can influence the effects that medications have on the body. Medications affect nutrition in four main areas. They can stimulate or suppress the appetite. They can alter the amount of nutrients absorbed and the rate of absorption. They affect the way the body breaks down and uses up nutrients. Finally, medications can slow down or speed up the rate at which food passes through the digestive tract.

Always ask your pediatrician, your pharmacist, and other specialists involved in your child's med-

ical care to explain whether medication should be taken with meals or on an empty stomach. Several antibiotics can cause stomach pain or upset unless taken with food. Also find out whether taking medication with a specific food, such as a glass of milk or orange juice, can make the treatment more or less effective, and ask what foods, if any, should be avoided during treatment.

Following are interactions seen between commonly used medications and foods, and guidelines for preventing such interactions or keeping the effects to a minimum.

Medication	Interactions with Nutrients	Dietary Guidelines
Antacids • Nonprescription indigestion remedies	Foods lessen effects.	Take 1 hour after eating.
Antibiotics In general	Reduce intestinal production of biotin (a B vitamin), pantothenic acid (vitamin B$_5$), and vitamin K; can speed up passage of food through intestine, decreasing availability for absorption.	Eat a well-balanced diet, including plenty of vegetables, grains, and cereals, to ensure adequate intake of all vitamins.
• Amoxicillin	Food slows absorption but does not alter dose effect.	None needed.
• Erythromycin stearate • Penicillin G/VK	Food decreases absorption.	Take 1 hour before or 2 hours after meals.
• Clarithromycin • Erythromycin estolate/succinate	Food improves absorption.	Take with meals.

• Tetracycline	Binds calcium and iron so that neither antibiotic nor mineral can be absorbed.	Take 2 hours before or after meals and other medications such as iron supplements or calcium-based antacids.
Anticonvulsant/antiepileptic medications • Phenobarbital • Phenytoin • Primidone	Interfere with vitamin D metabolism and thus with calcium absorption; also alter absorption of folic acid.	A good intake of vitamin D (found in fortified milk, egg yolks, oily fish, sunlight), calcium (dairy foods, leafy greens, broccoli, canned fish with bones), and folic acid (fresh fruits, vegetables, grains) should offset medication effects; ask your pediatrician about vitamin D and calcium supplements if your child is on long-term epilepsy treatment; folic acid supplements should not be used because overly high blood levels may decrease anticonvulsant efficacy.
• Phenytoin	Better absorbed with food or milk	Take with a meal or a glass of milk.
Antihistamines/decongestants • Chlorpheniramine • Oxymetazoline • Pseudoephedrine	Some medications given to relieve allergy or common cold symptoms may increase the appetite; effects and side effects may be increased by caffeine.	Provide ample servings of grains, cereals, fruits, and vegetables, low in fat and calories, to ensure a feeling of satisfaction without excessive calorie intake leading to unwanted weight gain; avoid caffeine-containing beverages such as coffee, tea, colas, and other soft drinks.
Nonsteroidal anti-inflammatory medications • Aspirin (acetylsalicylic acid)	Interferes with storage of vitamin C; may cause iron loss through bleeding in digestive tract.	Do not give aspirin to children because it has been associated with Reye syndrome, a rare but serious disease affecting the brain and liver following viral infections; use acetaminophen or ibuprofen unless your pediatrician specifically prescribes aspirin.

Asthma medications • Theophylline *(also see Antihistamines/Decongestants, above)*	Side effects more severe if taken with high-fat foods; anti-asthma effect reduced if dose coincides with consumption of charcoal-broiled foods; effects and side effects increased by caffeine.	Eat no more than 30 percent of daily calories in the form of fat, with saturated fat $1/3$ or less of total fat; avoid charcoal-broiled foods; avoid caffeine-containing drinks such as coffee, tea, colas, and other soft drinks.
Antituberculosis medications • Isoniazid	Interferes with vitamin B_6 (pyridoxine) metabolism.	Eat a well-balanced diet, including sources of vitamin B_6 such as grains, spinach, sweet and white potatoes, bananas, watermelon, prunes.
Corticosteroids • Prednisone • Hydrocortisone	May promote excretion of potassium and calcium.	Reduce salt intake; eat foods high in potassium (fresh fruits and vegetables) and calcium (low-fat dairy foods) to counter loss of these minerals.
Laxatives • Mineral oil	Interferes with the absorption of fat-soluble vitamins in the first part of the intestine.	Provide a diet rich in vegetables and fruits for fiber and encourage your child to drink plenty of water; if constipation is a problem, ask your pediatrician's advice. When mineral oil is prescribed, it should be given at bedtime, after most of the day's food has passed through the first part of the intestine.
Oral contraceptives • Various brands	Alter blood cholesterol levels; increase need for folic acid and vitamin B_6.	Use another form of contraception if there is a family history of high blood cholesterol or heart disease; consume plenty of fresh fruits and vegetables, grains and cereals, potatoes, and other sources of folic acid and vitamin B_6; take with food to prevent nausea.

Standard Growth Charts

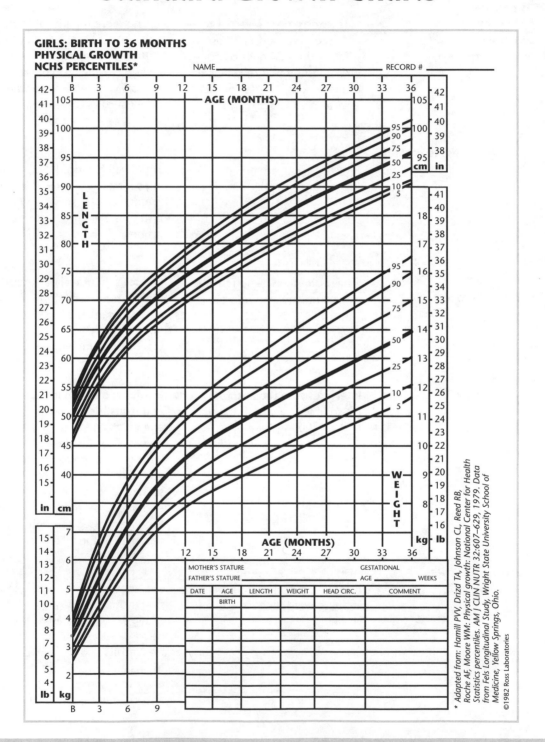

GIRLS: BIRTH TO 36 MONTHS
PHYSICAL GROWTH
NCHS PERCENTILES*

NAME _____ RECORD # _____

* Adapted from: Hamill PVV, Drizd TA, Johnson CL, Reed RB, Roche AF, Moore WM: Physical growth: National Center for Health Statistics percentiles. AM J CLIN NUTR 32:607–629, 1979. Data from Fels Longitudinal Study, Wright State University School of Medicine, Yellow Springs, Ohio.
©1982 Ross Laboratories

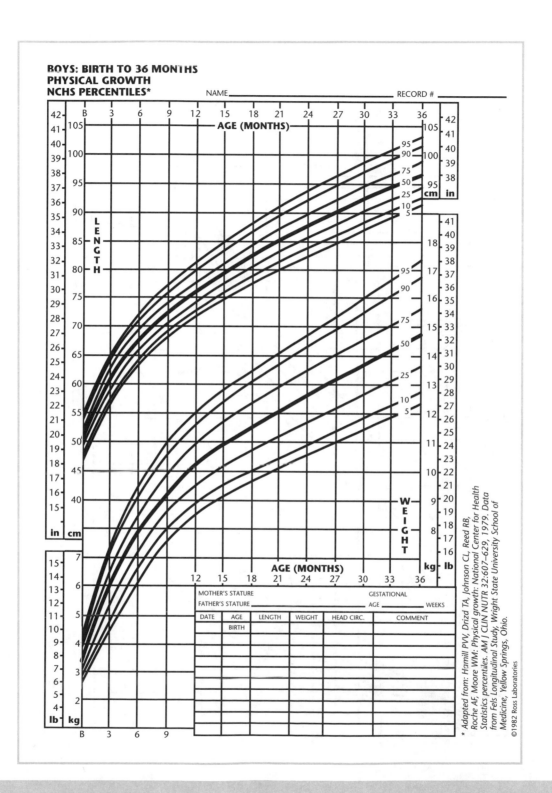

BOYS: BIRTH TO 36 MONTHS
PHYSICAL GROWTH
NCHS PERCENTILES*

NAME_____ RECORD #_____

AGE (MONTHS)

LENGTH

WEIGHT

AGE (MONTHS)

MOTHER'S STATURE   GESTATIONAL
FATHER'S STATURE _____ AGE _____ WEEKS

DATE	AGE	LENGTH	WEIGHT	HEAD CIRC.	COMMENT
	BIRTH				

* Adapted from: Hamill PVV, Drizd TA, Johnson CL, Reed RB, Roche AF, Moore WM: Physical growth: National Center for Health Statistics percentiles. AM J CLIN NUTR 32:607–629, 1979. Data from Fels Longitudinal Study, Wright State University School of Medicine, Yellow Springs, Ohio.
©1982 Ross Laboratories

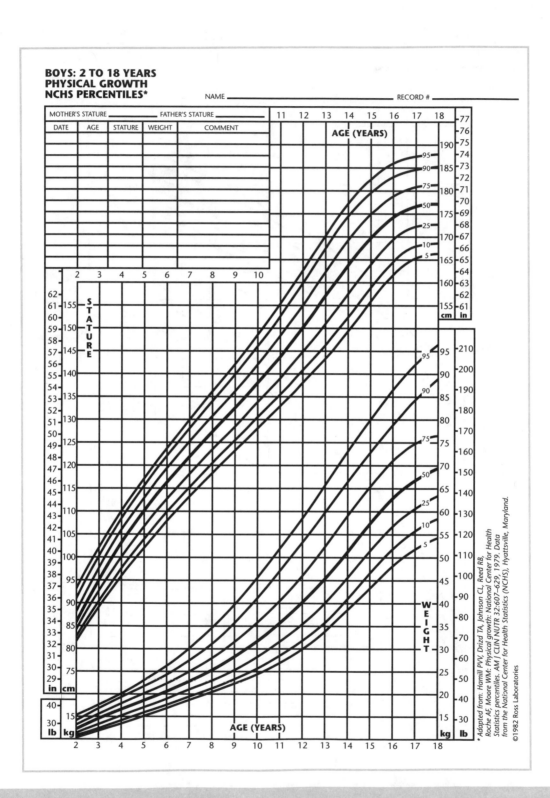

BOYS: 2 TO 18 YEARS
PHYSICAL GROWTH
NCHS PERCENTILES*

NAME _____ RECORD # _____

MOTHER'S STATURE _____ FATHER'S STATURE _____

DATE	AGE	STATURE	WEIGHT	COMMENT

AGE (YEARS)

STATURE

WEIGHT

AGE (YEARS)

* Adapted from: Hamill PVV, Drizd TA, Johnson CL, Reed RB, Roche AF, Moore WM: Physical growth: National Center for Health Statistics percentiles. AM J CLIN NUTR 32:607–629, 1979. Data from the National Center for Health Statistics (NCHS), Hyattsville, Maryland.

©1982 Ross Laboratories

GIRLS: 2 TO 18 YEARS
PHYSICAL GROWTH
NCHS PERCENTILES*

NAME _____ RECORD # _____

* Adapted from: Hamill PVV, Drizd TA, Johnson CL, Reed RB, Roche AF, Moore WM: Physical growth: National Center for Health Statistics percentiles. AM J CLIN NUTR 32:607–629, 1979. Data from the National Center for Health Statistics (NCHS), Hyattsville, Maryland.

©1982 Ross Laboratories

APPENDIX IV

Body Mass Index Charts

BODY MASS INDEX FOR SELECTED WEIGHTS AND STATURES*

Stature m (in)	1.24 (49)	1.27 (50)	1.30 (51)	1.32 (52)	1.35 (53)	1.37 (54)	1.40 (55)	1.42 (56)	1.45 (57)	1.47 (58)	1.50 (59)	1.52 (60)	1.55 (61)	1.57 (62)
Weight kg (lb)														
20 (45)	13	13	12	12	11	11	10	10	10	9	9	9	8	
23 (50)	15	14	13	13	12	12	12	11	11	10	10	10	9	9
25 (55)	16	15	15	14	14	13	13	12	12	12	11	11	10	10
27 (60)	18	17	16	16	15	15	14	13	13	13	12	12	11	11
29 (65)	19	18	17	17	16	16	15	15	14	14	13	13	12	12
32 (70)	21	20	19	18	17	17	16	16	15	15	14	14	13	13
34 (75)	22	21	20	20	19	18	17	17	16	16	15	15	14	14
36 (80)	24	22	21	21	20	19	19	18	17	17	16	16	15	15
39 (85)	25	24	23	22	21	21	20	19	18	18	17	17	16	16
41 (90)	27	25	24	23	22	22	21	20	19	19	18	18	17	17
43 (95)	28	27	25	25	24	23	22	21	20	20	19	19	18	17
45 (100)	29	28	27	26	25	24	23	22	22	21	20	20	19	18
48 (105)	31	30	28	27	26	25	24	24	23	22	21	21	20	19
50 (110)	32	31	30	29	27	27	25	25	24	23	22	22	21	20
52 (115)	34	32	31	30	29	28	27	26	25	24	23	23	22	21
54 (120)	35	34	32	31	30	29	28	27	26	25	24	24	23	22
57 (125)	37	35	34	33	31	30	29	28	27	26	25	25	24	23
59 (130)	38	37	35	34	32	31	30	29	28	27	26	26	25	24
61 (135)	40	38	36	35	34	33	31	30	29	28	27	27	25	25
64 (140)	41	39	38	36	35	34	32	31	30	29	28	27	26	26
66 (145)	43	41	39	38	36	35	34	33	31	30	29	28	27	27
68 (150)	44	42	40	39	37	36	35	34	32	31	30	29	28	28
70 (155)	46	44	42	40	39	37	36	35	33	33	31	30	29	29
73 (160)	47	45	43	42	40	39	37	35	35	34	32	31	30	29
77 (170)	50	48	46	44	42	41	39	38	37	36	34	33	32	31
79 (175)	...	49	47	46	44	42	40	39	38	37	35	34	33	32

BODY MASS INDEX FOR SELECTED WEIGHTS AND STATURES, CONTINUED

Stature m (in)	1.24 (49)	1.27 (50)	1.30 (51)	1.32 (52)	1.35 (53)	1.37 (54)	1.40 (55)	1.42 (56)	1.45 (57)	1.47 (58)	1.50 (59)	1.52 (60)	1.55 (61)	1.57 (62)
Weight kg (lb)														
82 (180)	...	51	48	47	45	44	42	40	39	38	36	35	34	33
84 (185)	...	...	50	48	46	45	43	42	40	39	37	36	35	34
86 (190)	...	...	...	49	47	46	44	43	41	40	39	37	36	35
88 (195)	...	...	...	51	49	47	45	44	42	41	39	38	37	36
91 (200)	...	...	...	...	50	48	46	45	43	42	40	39	38	37
93 (205)	...	...	...	...	...	50	47	46	44	43	41	40	39	38
95 (210)	...	...	...	...	...	...	49	47	45	44	42	41	40	39
98 (215)	...	...	...	...	...	...	50	48	46	45	43	42	41	40
100 (220)	...	...	...	...	...	...	...	49	47	46	44	43	42	40
102 (225)	...	...	...	...	...	...	...	51	49	47	45	44	42	41
104 (230)	...	...	...	...	...	...	...	...	50	48	46	45	43	42
107 (235)	...	...	...	...	...	...	...	...	...	49	47	46	44	43
109 (240)	...	...	...	...	...	...	...	...	...	50	48	47	45	44
111 (245)	...	...	...	...	...	...	...	...	...	...	49	48	46	45
113 (250)	...	...	...	...	...	...	...	...	...	...	50	49	47	46
116 (255)	...	...	...	...	...	...	...	...	...	...	...	50	48	47
118 (260)	...	...	...	...	...	...	...	...	...	...	...	...	49	48
120 (265)	...	...	...	...	...	...	...	...	...	...	...	...	50	49
122 (270)	...	...	...	...	...	...	...	...	...	...	...	...	...	50
125 (275)	...	...	...	...	...	...	...	...	...	...	...	...	...	...
127 (280)	...	...	...	...	...	...	...	...	...	...	...	...	...	...
129 (285)	...	...	...	...	...	...	...	...	...	...	...	...	...	...
132 (290)	...	...	...	...	...	...	...	...	...	...	...	...	...	...
134 (295)	...	...	...	...	...	...	...	...	...	...	...	...	...	...
136 (300)	...	...	...	...	...	...	...	...	...	...	...	...	...	...

BODY MASS INDEX FOR SELECTED WEIGHTS AND STATURES, CONTINUED

Stature m (in)	1.60 (63)	1.63 (64)	1.65 (65)	1.68 (66)	1.70 (67)	1.73 (68)	1.75 (69)	1.78 (70)	1.80 (71)	1.83 (72)	1.85 (73)	1.88 (74)	1.90 (75)	1.93 (76)
Weight kg (lb)														
20 (45)	9	9	8	...	...	...	...	...	...	...	...	...	...	...
25 (50)	10	9	9	9	...	...	...	...	...	...	...	...	...	...
27 (55)	11	10	10	10	9	9	...	...	...	...	...	...	...	...
29 (65)	12	11	11	10	10	10	10	...	...	...	...	...	...	...
32 (70)	12	12	12	11	11	11	10	10	...	...	...	...	...	...
34 (75)	13	13	12	12	12	11	11	11	10	...	...	...	...	...
36 (80)	14	14	13	13	13	12	12	11	11	11	...	...	...	...
39 (85)	15	15	14	14	13	13	13	12	12	12	11	...	...	...
41 (90)	16	15	15	14	14	14	13	13	13	12	12	12	...	...
43 (95)	17	16	16	15	15	14	14	13	13	13	12	12	...	...
45 (100)	18	17	17	16	16	15	15	14	14	14	13	13	13	12
48 (105)	19	18	17	17	16	16	16	15	15	14	14	13	13	13
50 (110)	19	19	18	18	17	17	16	16	16	15	15	14	14	13
52 (115)	20	20	19	18	18	17	17	16	16	16	15	15	14	14
54 (120)	21	20	20	19	19	18	18	17	17	16	16	15	15	15
57 (125)	22	21	21	20	20	19	19	18	17	17	17	16	16	15
59 (130)	23	22	22	21	20	20	19	19	18	18	17	17	16	16
61 (135)	24	23	22	22	21	20	20	19	19	18	18	17	17	16
64 (140)	25	24	23	22	22	21	21	20	20	19	19	18	18	17
66 (145)	26	25	24	23	23	22	21	21	20	20	19	19	18	18
68 (150)	27	26	25	24	24	23	22	21	21	20	20	19	19	18
70 (155)	27	26	26	25	24	23	23	22	22	21	21	20	19	19
73 (160)	28	27	27	26	25	24	24	23	22	22	21	21	20	19
77 (170)	30	29	28	27	27	26	25	24	24	23	23	22	21	21

BODY MASS INDEX FOR SELECTED WEIGHTS AND STATURES, CONTINUED

Stature m (in)	1.60 (63)	1.63 (64)	1.65 (65)	1.68 (66)	1.70 (67)	1.73 (68)	1.75 (69)	1.78 (70)	1.80 (71)	1.83 (72)	1.85 (73)	1.88 (74)	1.90 (75)	1.93 (76)
Weight kg (lb)														
82 (180)	32	31	30	29	28	27	27	26	25	24	24	23	23	22
84 (185)	33	32	31	30	29	28	27	26	26	25	25	24	23	23
86 (190)	34	32	32	31	30	29	28	27	27	26	25	24	24	23
88 (195)	35	33	32	31	31	30	29	28	27	26	26	25	25	24
91 (200)	35	34	33	32	31	30	30	29	28	27	27	26	25	24
93 (205)	36	35	34	33	32	31	30	29	29	28	27	26	26	25
95 (210)	37	36	35	34	33	32	31	30	29	28	28	27	26	26
98 (215)	38	37	36	35	34	33	32	31	30	29	28	28	27	26
100 (220)	39	38	37	35	35	33	33	31	31	30	29	28	28	27
102 (225)	40	38	37	36	35	34	33	32	31	30	30	29	28	27
104 (230)	41	39	38	37	36	35	34	33	32	31	30	30	29	28
107 (235)	42	40	39	38	37	36	35	34	33	32	31	30	30	29
109 (240)	43	41	40	39	38	36	36	34	34	33	32	31	30	29
111 (245)	43	42	41	39	38	37	36	35	34	33	32	31	31	30
113 (250)	44	43	42	40	39	38	37	36	35	34	33	32	31	30
116 (255)	45	44	42	41	40	39	38	37	36	35	34	33	32	31
118 (260)	46	44	43	42	41	39	39	37	36	35	34	33	33	32
120 (265)	47	45	44	43	42	40	39	38	37	36	35	34	33	32
122 (270)	48	46	45	43	42	41	40	39	38	37	36	35	34	33
125 (275)	49	47	46	44	43	42	41	39	38	37	36	35	35	33
127 (280)	50	48	47	45	44	42	41	40	39	38	37	36	35	34
129 (285)	50	49	47	46	45	43	42	41	40	39	38	37	36	35
132 (290)	...	50	48	47	46	44	43	42	41	39	38	37	36	35
134 (295)	...	50	49	47	46	45	44	42	41	40	39	38	37	36
136 (300)	...	...	50	48	47	45	44	43	42	41	40	39	38	37

*Reprinted by permission from *Guidelines for Adolescent Preventive Services (GAPS), Clinical Evaluation and Management Handbook*. Chicago, IL: American Medical Association; 1995. Copyright 1995, American Medical Association.

Food Substitutions

If your child won't eat:	Substitute:
Fruit	Vegetables, raw or cooked; if your child won't eat fresh fruits, try dried fruits such as apricots, pears, raisins, cherries, mango, pineapple, and bananas, and gradually introduce fresh fruits; make puréed sauces for yogurt with fresh or frozen fruit and gradually introduce chunks of whole fruit; serve applesauce instead of whole fruit. If your child refuses citrus fruits, offer alternative sources of vitamin C (strawberries, cantaloupe, vitamin C-enriched juices, broccoli and other cruciferous vegetables, watermelon, potatoes, etc.); try mixing fruits such as blueberries, chopped apples, and bananas in muffin, quickbread, and waffle batters.
Meat	Fish, poultry, eggs, tofu, legumes (dried beans, chickpeas, and peas) and grains, and peanut butter; use chopped vegetable mixtures instead of ground meat or poultry to make pasta sauces, taco fillings, etc.; breads, crackers, and pasta made with iron-fortified flour.
Milk	Cheeses, yogurts, and other dairy foods made with cow's, goat's, or sheep's milk; soy- and rice-based substitutes for milk and cheese (ask your pediatrician whether your child should be taking supplements of vitamins B_{12} and D); canned fish with bones (salmon, sardines, herring) for calcium and vitamin D; good vegetable sources of calcium such as broccoli; safe exposure to sunlight for vitamin D.
Vegetables	If your child refuses green leafy vegetables, try dark yellow and orange vegetables (carrots, squash, sweet potatoes) for vitamin A and folic acid, fruits and fruit juices for vitamin C, as well as folic acid; a child who turns down cooked vegetables may enjoy raw vegetable sticks and salads; offer low-sodium vegetable juice instead of fruit juice; children who balk at plain vegetables may enjoy Asian-style stir-fried vegetables; make pasta and taco sauces with finely chopped vegetables instead of, or in addition to, meat.
Whole-grain breads	High-fiber white bread; whole-wheat and rye crackers; whole-wheat pasta.

Health and Nutritional Resources

ALLERGIES AND ASTHMA

**Allergy and Asthma Network/
Mothers of Asthmatics Inc.**
2751 Prosperity Avenue
Suite 150
Fairfax, VA 22031
(703) 641-9595
(800) 878-4403

**The Asthma and Allergy Foundation
of America**
1125 15th Street, NW
Suite 502
Washington, DC 20005
(800) 7-ASTHMA

**National Institute of Allergy and
Infectious Disease**
Office of Communications
Building 31, Room 7A-50
9000 Rockville Pike
Bethesda, MD 20892
(301) 496-5717

**National Heart, Lung and
Blood Institute**
Asthma Prevention
National Institutes of Health
P.O. Box 30105
Bethesda, MD 20824-0105
(301) 251-1222

The Food Allergy Network
10400 Eaton Place
Suite 107
Fairfax, VA 22030
(703) 691-3179

BREASTFEEDING

La Leche League International
1400 North Meacham Road
Schaumburg, IL 60173-4840
(800) LA LECHE
(847) 519-7730

DIABETES

Juvenile Diabetes Foundation
432 Park Avenue South
New York, NY 10016
(800) 223-1138

DIGESTIVE DISORDERS

**Crohn's Disease &
Colitis Foundation of America**
386 Park Avenue South
New York, NY 10016
(800) 932-2423 (information)
(800) 343-3637 (literature)

**National Digestive Diseases
Information Clearinghouse**
2 Information Way
Bethesda, MD 20892-3570
(301) 654-3810

EATING DISORDERS

**American Anorexia/Bulimia Association Inc.
(AABA)**
165 West 46th Street
Suite 1108
New York NY 10036
(212) 575-6200

Center for the Study of Anorexia and Bulimia
1841 Broadway
New York, NY 10023
(212) 333-3444

GLUTEN ENTEROPATHY/CELIAC DISEASE
Gluten Intolerance Group of North America
P.O. Box 23053
Seattle, WA 98102-0353
(206) 325-6980

Celiac Disease Foundation
13251 Ventura Blvd., Suite 1
Studio City, CA 91604-1838
(818) 990-2354

Celiac Sprue Association/USA Inc.
P.O. Box 31700
Omaha, NE 68131-0700
(402) 558-0600

Resources from the American Academy of Pediatrics

The American Academy of Pediatrics develops and produces a wide variety of public education materials that teach parents and children the importance of preventive and therapeutic medical care. These materials include books, magazines, videos, brochures, and other educational resources. Examples of these materials include:

- Brochures and fact sheets on allergies, child-care issues, divorce and single parenting, growth and development, immunizations, learning disabilities, nutrition and fitness, sleep problems, substance abuse, and television.
- Videos on immunizations, newborn care, nutrition education, and asthma.
- First aid and growth charts, child health records, and books for parents.

For a copy of the Academy's Parents Resource Guide, send a self-addressed, stamped no. 10 envelope to:

American Academy of Pediatrics
Department PRG
PO Box 927
Elk Grove Village, IL 60009-0927

For help finding a qualified pediatrician or pediatric subspecialist, contact the "Pediatrician Referral Source" of the American Academy of Pediatrics by sending the name of your town (or those nearby) and a self-addressed, stamped envelope to:

American Academy of Pediatrics
Pediatrician Referral
PO Box 927
Elk Grove Village, IL 60009-0927

The standard growth charts and body mass index tables in Appendices III and IV have been revised by the National Center for Health Statistics and the Centers for Disease Control since this book went to press. To obtain the revised charts and tables, please write to the Academy or contact our website at http:// www.aap.org.

Index

high-protein for infants, 25

to introduce solid foods, 24

Cesarean section, breastfeeding position, 8

Cheese, and dental health, 171

and lactose intolerance, 114

Chewing ability, 24, 42, 46, 109

Childcare, group, and gastroenteritis, 113

and picky eating, 66

Chloride, 103, 120, 154.

See also Electrolytes.

Chocolate and dental health, 171

Choking, first aid, 48

and solid foods, 29

and pouching, 49, 109-110

in breastfed infant, 18

risks in toddlers, 42, 46-47

Cholesterol, acceptable levels, 166

in adopted children, 166

reducing, 166-167

testing, 166

Cholesterol-lowering medications, 168

American Academy of Pediatrics recommendations, 168

Cleft lip/palate, 18

Clostridium botulinum. See Botulism.

Colic, 16-17

and picky eating, 65

Colitis. *See* Inflammatory bowel disease.

Computer games, **American Academy of Pediatrics recommended limit, 134**

Constipation, and acne, 86

and irritable bowel syndrome, 117

after viral illness, 64

in eating disorders, 121, 148

in infants, 17

in school-age children, 64-65

Corn allergy, 200

Cow's milk, allergy, 198

American Academy of Pediatrics recommendations, 169

and allergies in infants, 20

and constipation, 121

damages intestine, 12

in infants, 12

Crash diets. *See* Weight loss.

Crohn disease, *See* Inflammatory bowel disease.

Cystic fibrosis, 120-121

D

Dairy foods, low consumption by adolescent girls, 72, 77

Dehydration, and diabetes, 169

and eating disorders, 81, 148

in chronic diseases, 81

in infant, 17

prevention, 64, 94, 103, 110

thirst not a guide, 81

Dental health. *See* Nursing-bottle caries, Tooth decay.

Desserts, and misguided control of food intake, 40

for infants, 40

Diabetes, 168-169

Diapers, guide to infant feeding, 16

Diarrhea, 113-117

and childcare, 173

and cooked apples, 65

and gluten enteropathy, 119

and irritable bowel syndrome, 117

and juice, 33

and sugar, 110, 117

in infants, 17

in toddler, 45

normal diet, 117

vs. stool retention, 120

See also Toddler diarrhea

Diet fads, 148

Hirschsprung disease, 119

Histamine, 198

Home-made foods for infants. *See* Infant foods.

Honey, and tooth decay, 171

> **American Academy of Pediatrics
> recommendation:** unsafe for infants, 31

Hormonal problems, and
overweight, 126

Human immunodeficiency virus/HIV, 6

Hunger, inborn signal, 65
stimulus to eat, 38, 44

Hyperactivity, 178, 192-193, 204

I

Ileitis. *See* Inflammatory bowel disease.

Immune system, and food allergies, 26

Immunization, 180

Infant feeding, changing views, 19

Infant foods, mixed, 32, 34
commercial, 30-32
desserts, 35
dinners, 35
freezing, 32
home-made, 30
organic, 31
safe preparation, 30

Infectious diseases, and
breastfeeding, 14

Inflammatory bowel disease, 118

Intolerance, food.
See Food intolerance.

Intolerance, lactose.
See Lactose intolerance.

Iron, absorption rate, 75, 91, 104
athletes' needs, 75
-deficiency anemia, 74, 104
deficiency in adolescents, 74-75, 104
fortified cereal for babies, 33-34, 104

heme, nonheme, 75
in adolescent diet, 74
in alternative diets, 189
risk of excessive intake, 33
sources, 34, 75
stores in infant, 25, 104

Irradiation of food, 182

Irritable bowel syndrome, 117-118

Isatin, 65, 122

J

Jaundice and breastfeeding, 17-18

Juice, and diarrhea, 45
causing rash, 204
for babies, 33
unpasteurized, 34
vegetable, 34

See also Fruit, Toddler Diarrhea.

K

Ketogenic diet, 193

L

Lactation consultant, 6, 13

Lacto-ovo-vegetarian diet, 188

Lacto-vegetarian diet, 188

Lactose, and calcium absorption, 103
-free milk/dairy products, 117
hidden sources, 201
intolerance, 114, 118-119, 201-202

Laxatives, 121

Leaky breasts. *See* Breastfeeding problem solving.

Leftovers, and food safety, 176
in baby bottles, 13
school lunches, 63
solid foods, 30, 32

Rice cereal for infants, 24, 203
Rooting reflex, 7, 18
Rumination, 109

S

Safety tips for food preparation, 32, 116, 173-175
Salt, in infant foods, 30
    in normal diet, 103, 154
See also Salt pills.
Salt pills, 82, 103
School lunches, 60-63, 157
    National School Lunch Program, 61
    Team Nutrition, 61
    School Meals Initiative for Healthy Children, 61
Seizures, 193
Selenium, 121
Self-feeding, in infants, 28-29
    in toddlers, 40
Sensitive mouth.
    See Oral sensitivity.
Serotonin, 82
Serving sizes, Food Guide Pyramid, 89-90, 92
    for adolescents, 75
    for infants, 25, 30, 32
    for toddlers, 41-42
    fruit juice, 33
    vegetables, 92
Sexual activity/arousal, and acne, 85
    and breastfeeding, 15, 19
Sexual maturation. *See* Puberty.
Sham feeding, 66
Short-order cooking, 38-39, 53
Sleep apnea, 132
Sleepovers, 54
Sleepy baby, and feeding
    problems, 17
Smoking, and children's health risks, 169
    and fat distribution, 86

See also Nicotine.
Snacks, for school-age athletes, 64
    for toddlers, 42-43
    not in front of TV, 46, 126
    unrestricted, 65
Sodium. *See* Salt, Electrolytes.
Solid foods/feeding,
    acceptance, 27
    **American Academy of Pediatrics
        recommendations, 23**
    and breastfeeding, 23, 26
    and constipation, 121
    and sleep, 25
    and water, 16
    baby's position, 27
    consistency, 24
    father's involvement, 25
    guidelines for introduction, 28
    in bottles, 26, 107
    readiness, 23-24
Sorbitol, 45, 65, 115, 122, 200
Soy intolerance/allergy, 119, 199
Spastic colon. *See* Irritable bowel syndrome.
Spitting up, 16, 107
See also Gastroesophageal reflux.
Sports, 64, 81
See also Sports drinks.
Sports drinks, 64, 82, 110, 113, 117
Standard growth charts, 127
Sterilizing bottles/nipples, 12-13.
Starches. *See* Carbohydrates.
Steroids, anabolic, 78
Stool(s), in infants, 17, 33
retention, 120
See also Bowel movements, Constipation, Diarrhea,
    Toddler diarrhea.
Strength training, 79
Stress, and vomiting, 111
Sugar, and diarrhea, 110, 113